EXPERIMENTS IN
GENERAL AND BIOMEDICAL INSTRUMENTATION

MORRIS TISCHLER

**President, OMG Techsource Company and
Career Education Associates, Inc.**

McGraw-Hill Book Company
Gregg Division

New York   Atlanta   Dallas   St. Louis   San Francisco   Auckland
Bogotá   Düsseldorf   Johannesburg   London   Madrid   Mexico
Montreal   New Delhi   Panama   Paris   São Paulo   Singapore
Sydney   Tokyo   Toronto

Sponsoring Editor Mark Haas
Editing Supervisor Karen Sekiguchi
Design Supervisors Tracy Glasner, Caryl Valerie Spinka
Production Supervisor Priscilla Taguer
Art Supervisor George T. Resch

Cover Designer A Good Thing, Inc.
Technical Studio Burmar Technical Corp.

Linear Integrated Circuit Applications Series:

Experiments in Amplifiers, Filters, Oscillators, and Generators

Experiments in Telecommunications

Experiments in General and Biomedical Instrumentation

ISBN 0-07-064781-X

1 2 3 4 5 6 7 8 9 0   SMSM   8 8 7 6 5 4 3 2 1 0

CONTENTS

Preface

Most modern electronic circuitry incorporates high-density packaging in the form of linear and/or digital integrated circuit chips (ICs). Radios, TV sets, medical instruments, citizen band radios, calculators, and computers are but a few examples of equipment which uses high-density packaging of solid-state devices. During the 1960s, the study of linear circuits used in operational amplifiers (op amps) and analog computers was left to the area of "nice-to-know" information, in favor of teaching the digital circuitry used in computer logic. Although linear IC technology stands today where transistors stood in the 1950s, the renewed use of the basic op amp design and its myriad variations now make linear devices as important as digital devices to the electronics technician.

The *Linear Integrated Circuits Applications Series* is aimed at presenting linear ICs in a variety of circuit applications. Linear ICs are easy to teach and even easier to learn. In the application of the devices there are no load lines to plot, no calculations using complex parameters, and a minimum of biasing problems. In laboratory usage, an important consideration is that most linear chips are rugged and not easily burned out. Low cost, a wide variety of types, and ease in handling make linear ICs very appealing for the designer. As prerequisites for studying linear ICs the student needs only DC, AC, and the general concepts of active devices. A brief course in transistor theory is sufficient since such information is not essential for working with ICs. The key in using chips is knowing how to apply them in circuit designs.

In each volume of this series the introduction of a new chip includes a discussion about the chip. For instructional purposes, only those chips which provide for a wide range of applications were selected. The cost of the chips to the student was also considered in selecting those used in these experiments. The laboratory instruments and components required for circuit evaluation are described in each text-lab manual. In most cases ¼-or 1/10-W resistors are adequate and 10 percent capacitors with 25 W V DC ratings will be adequate. All required components needed for a circuit are shown on the circuit diagrams. The text-manual is not written in cookbook fashion. The student should know how to use electronic components, how to wire circuits, and should be experienced in the use of general types of laboratory instruments. Three instruments are particularly important, namely, a dual-trace oscilloscope, a functions generator, and a digital multimeter.

The study of linear integrated circuits and their applications is challenging and provides ample opportunity for students to express their creative ability. Students completing the study will have a thorough knowledge in the use, application, and methods of troubleshooting electronic circuits that incorporate linear ICs in their design.

ACKNOWLEDGMENTS

Acknowledgment is given to John L. Sheppard for his assistance in validating the experiments; to John S. Taylor and Dr. Prem J. Bhatt for reviewing the manuscripts; to Joseph Werner for the artwork and original layout; to Thomas D. Evans for bringing the units of study and materials together; to Esther M. Scheffel and Beverly Siegel for typing; to Alan Siegel, Lewis Siegel, and Joanne S. Tischler for their efforts in collating the manuscript. All are members of OMG Techsource Company.

Special mention is given to my favorite co-worker and beautiful wife, Maureen S. Tischler, who made an enormous effort in proofing, arranging, and bringing the material into final form.

Acknowledgment is also given to various component manufacturers who contributed their technical data. Particular recognition is given to Motorola, National Semiconductor, RCA, Texas Instruments, Fairchild, Signetics, and General Instrument Company. Finally, mention is made of Ruth J. Tischler, my late wife, whose passing caused me to return to my workbench to design, experiment, and write in order to find myself.

INTRODUCTION

GENERAL OBJECTIVES

Upon completion of this course of study and when provided with circuit diagrams using linear integrated circuits (ICs) as well as laboratory test instruments, you will be able to:

1. *Measure circuit voltages and waveshapes and compare them with the data provided*
2. *Troubleshoot electronic circuits and replace defective parts*
3. *Assemble and test electronic circuits using linear ICs and vary component values to derive desired results*
4. *Develop electronic circuits within the range of subjects covered by this course in order to meet specific requirements*
5. *Use electronic laboratory test instruments to measure voltages, waveshapes, phase relationship, distortion, and frequencies in order to determine the circuit's operating characteristics*
6. *Use data sheets for integrated circuits in order to determine which components should be used in circuit development or replaced during repair*
7. *Handle sensitive components, such as ICs, during installation and repair without damaging parts*
8. *Discuss with other engineers and technicians the operation of circuits and subsystems as covered in this course*
9. *Determine the limitation of test instruments used in electronic measurements and troubleshooting*
10. *Write technical reports relating to circuit development, repair, or maintenance and describing the circuit, the operating values, the malfunction, and the repair performed*

GENERAL INTRODUCTION

Electronics is fascinating because the individual has many opportunities to be creative and find solutions to electronic problems. Each new and seemingly complex piece of equipment can be divided into a series of basic circuits which use relatively few different types of electronic components. One component, such as a tube, transistor, or integrated circuit, can be wired so as to perform numerous functions. This text-manual provides for the application of linear ICs in an array of electronic circuits.

This course does not use a "cookbook" approach, wherein you would be given step-by-step details; rather, the instructions are purposely brief, with only the general idea conveyed, thus leaving the thinking to you, the learner.

Each circuit is to be studied in order to determine how it functions. Indeed, the circuit may not perform properly when it is first connected—all the more fun! A circuit that does not work promptly requires more thinking, testing, changing of component values, and so on. If you are a highly qualified technician or an engineer, you need only the circuit concept and basic information in order to get started. From this starting point plus your test instruments, you should be able to make a functional circuit.

Some circuits are provided with equations to enable you to make your own calculations and circuit changes. Some tests are required, and others may be suggested by either the instructor or you, the student. At all times you should be saying to yourself, "What if . . . I changed the bias, varied the voltage, increased the load? What would happen?" The "what if" provides a greater insight into circuit design.

Several circuits can be combined to form subsystems. You may want to consider the design, the assembly, and the testing of such configurations and then combine the new subsystems to form larger operating entities. It is suggested that a brief laboratory report be prepared on each circuit studied. The format of the report should be determined by the electronics instructor.

The circuits to be studied will require certain laboratory test instruments. The following types should be available:

Oscilloscope, 5-in, dual-trace, triggered sweep
Function generator, sine wave, triangular wave, and square wave, 1 hertz (Hz) to 1 megahertz (MHz)
Digital multimeter and field-effect-transistor volt-ohm-milliammeter (FETVOM)
Capacitance and/or *RCL* bridge

1

Resistance and capacitance decade substitution boxes
Grid-dip meter [for radio-frequency (RF) circuits only]
Distortion meter or analyzer (optional)

Appropriate instrument test leads, probes, and alligator jumpers are also required. An electronic calculator will be a time-saver and should be available, for calculations are required in circuit changes. The parts required for each circuit are shown on the circuit diagrams. Resistors are all ¼ watt (W) unless otherwise indicated. Capacitors are rated at 25 W V DC (working volts of direct current).

A word of advice. When you design or redesign a circuit, think about how you would change it if the circuit didn't perform as expected. Consider several alternatives. Try your circuit, try it again, and retry it until your idea is converted into a working circuit or system.

SUGGESTED LABORATORY INSTRUMENTS

Various types and qualities of electronic test instruments are available. Obviously, an oscilloscope that sells for over $2000 is better and probably more professional than one which sells for $400 to $700. Such expensive instruments can be used but are not required for this course of study. The instruments mentioned in the sections that follow will perform adequately.

Laboratory Power Supply

To perform the experiments, well-regulated power supplies are required. A well-regulated dual floating power supply with $\pm$ 20 V DC at 0.1 ampere (A), and $+5$ V at 0.1 A is required. The 20-V sources should be adjustable, and the ripple should be less than 10 millivolts (mV) with full load.

Oscilloscope

A 5-in, dual-trace, triggered-sweep oscilloscope should be used. It should be equipped with:

Vertical sensitivity, 10 mV/cm each channel, frequency response DC to 15 MHz, with DC and alternating current (AC) input
Horizontal 200 mV/cm, frequency responses 2 to 200 kHz
Sweep speed, 1 microsecond per centimeter (μs/cm) to 0.2 μs/cm
Magnification, $\times$10
Two probes, direct and one $\times$10 attenuation
Test leads (optional)

Function Generator

This instrument should have a frequency range of 1 Hz to 2 MHz, with less than 0.1 percent distortion for sine waves, triangular waves, and square waves. The stepped and variable attenuation should be 0 to 60 dB, with 10-V output into a 50-Ω load.

Voltmeter

The digital multimeter is a most important instrument. It is suggested that a VOM or FETVOM be available along with a digital multimeter since two measurements may sometimes be needed simultaneously. Many different types of digital multimeter are available.

Impedance Bridge

A capacitance of *RCL* bridge (one or two per laboratory) will be useful for checking component values since, for instance, a capacitor market 20 μF may actually measure 25 μF or more (20 percent tolerance value). The unit should measure resistance at 0.001 to 11 MΩ, capacitance 1 pF to 11,000 μF, inductance from .01 μH to 1100 H, battery and AC operated.

Resistance-Capacitance Decade Boxes

At least one each of these boxes should be available per work station since it is often more convenient to vary the resistance or capacitance value by turning a knob than by inserting separate components. The suggested resistance decade box is 15 Ω to 10 MΩ in two ranges.

Distortion Meter

This instrument is used to measure the distortion of amplifiers. Usually one or two distortion meters per laboratory is sufficient. The instrument should be able to measure to within 0.1 percent and have a frequency range of 20 Hz to 20 kHz, distortion range of 0.3 to 100 percent, and input level of 1 to 300 V.

Grid-dip Meter

This instrument is used for measurements on RF circuits, and the suggested range is 1.5 to 250 MHz. One or two grid-dip meters per laboratory is sufficient.

Digital Frequency Counter (Optional)

This instrument should have a frequency range of 10 Hz to 60 MHz, sensitivity of 30 mV, and six-digit readout. One digital frequency counter per laboratory is sufficient.

LABORATORY EXPERIMENTS

A variety of construction projects for experimentation can be designed. Heat, light, and/or pulse detectors are typical circuits which can be constructed, tested, and evaluated. The materials required, equations, and test procedures are included in each experiment. Technical information on the chips used is found in Appendix A. For additional information, application notes from such component manufacturers as Motorola, Texas Instruments, National Semiconductor, and Fairchild should also be referred to. Construct the circuit and make suggested tests. Prepare a brief report and include the circuit developed and parameters listed.

There are many types of integrated circuits to select

from, and some are designed for specific applications. In this course, in order to economize, the ICs suggested are used to test circuit operations even though more specialized IC chips may exist, may be more effective, and may use fewer discrete components.

A few basic circuits have been selected. The same components, with possibly a few additions, can be used for variations of the circuits provided or in the study of many other types of circuits. Additional circuits are obtainable from data manuals listed in the bibliography. A set of these data manuals, which are nominal in cost, should be available for both student and instructor use. Data sheets for all solid-state devices provided in the components kit have been included in the Appendix. Laboratory exercises and related classroom discussions entail 50 to 75 h, or sometimes even 100 h, of activity.

Laboratory experiments call for specific types of measurement that require the use of test equipment. You may not be familiar with the methods of application of this equipment; thus you may seek instructor assistance or establish your own procedures. As an example, bandwidth (BW) measurements may be required on an audio amplifier. This calls for the audio generator source to be held at constant voltage and the amplifier output voltage monitored with a meter while the frequency is varied from 10 Hz to 20,000 Hz or higher. The resultant data, visually collected in octaves, should be plotted on semilogarithmic graph paper. For example, the output-input phase relationship of an amplifier can most easily be determined by connecting the input signal to the amplifier into the oscilloscope's horizontal input. A Lissajous pattern will be produced, from which the phase angle can be derived when the amplifier's output is connected to the scope's vertical input.

Technical Data

Technical data on ICs and circuits are provided in the Appendix. Armed with this information, you will be able not only to better understand the circuits under study, but also to design your own additional circuits.

Laboratory Experimentation Time

Each laboratory assignment will require at least two 2 hours for construction, testing and evaluation of the circuit. It is suggested that only the technical data be gathered and that the laboratory report be written outside the laboratory.

MATERIALS REQUIRED

The components are standard commercial- and industrial-grade parts which are available at most electronic parts outlets. The criteria for selection of these components are that they be available, of good quality, and of a size that could be easily handled by the experimenter. These components are given in the list that follows.

Component Tolerances

Generally, resistors of 5 percent or 10 percent tolerance can be used. Capacitors may be 10 to 20 percent tolerant or more. In circuits where matched pairs of components are needed, you should check your component values and try to match them as closely as possible. While 1 percent and 0.1 percent components are available, they are quite costly. Besides, it is good experience to learn when and how to find closely matching components from a low-tolerance batch since this is often necessary in fieldwork.

SOLID-STATE DEVICES:

1 LM324 IC	1 SN7402 IC
1 MC1496P IC	1 LM556 IC
1 LM339AN IC	1 SN7404 IC
1 LM3900N IC	1 LM565CN IC
1 LM375N IC	1 CA3051 IC
1 SN7400 IC	1 LM556 IC
1 LM552D IC	2 MC1495 ICs
1 MC3403P (or TL074) IC	

2 IN60 diodes
2 IN914 diodes
2 IN4733 Zener diodes
1 IN963 Zener diode
3 2N3904 NPN transistor
1 2N3905 PNP transistor
1 2N4871 unijunction transistor
3 2N5457 FET transistors
1 2N3638A transistor

RESISTORS (carbon composition 1/4 W, 10%):

1 47 Ω	1 2.2 MΩ
2 2.7 kΩ	8 1 kΩ
2 33 kΩ	1 18 kΩ
1 330 kΩ	2 270 kΩ
2 100 Ω	3 4.7 MΩ
3 3.3 kΩ	1 1.5 kΩ
3 47 kΩ	3 22 kΩ
3 470 kΩ	3 10 MΩ
2 150 Ω	3 2.2 kΩ
3 4.7 kΩ	1 27 kΩ
3 68 kΩ	
1 820 kΩ	
2 270 Ω	
2 8.2 kΩ	
7 100 kΩ	
4 1 MΩ	
3 330 Ω	
4 6.8 kΩ	
2 150 kΩ	
1 1.5 MΩ	
1 470 Ω	
8 10 kΩ	
1 180 kΩ	
1 6.8 MΩ	
3 680 Ω	
1 15 kΩ	
4 220 kΩ	

CAPACITORS: Working voltages of at least 25 V DC are satisfactory

Dipped silvered mica

1	10 pF 5%	1	100 pF 5%
3	15 pF 5%	1	150 pF 5%
1	30 pF 5%	1	270 pF 5%
1	47 pF 5%	2	330 pF 5%

Ceramic disc

1	470 pF 10%	3	0.005 μF 10%
2	680 pF 10%	6	0.01 μF 20%
3	0.001 μF 10%	4	0.02 μF 20%
3	0.002 μF 10%	4	0.05 μF 20%
4	0.003 μF 10%		

Mylar rectangular

7 0.1 μF 10%
2 0.2 μF 10%

Metalized Mylar

1 0.47 μF 10%

Electrolytic

6 1 μF −10 + 75%
4 5 μF −10 + 75%
2 10 μF −10 + 75%
1 25 μF −10 + 75%
2 50 μF −10 + 75%

Electrolytic single-ended

4 100 μF 20 to 30%

MISCELLANEOUS COMPONENTS:

3 500 μF 20 to 30% Electrolytic single-ended
4 14-pin IC sockets
1 Patching panel
2 10-kΩ potentiometers
1 4-in wire, 22 gauge Solid hook-up
2 100-kΩ potentiometers
1 loudspeaker, 8Ω
2 1-MΩ potentiometers
1 double-pole, double-throw push button, n.o. (DPDT) switches
1 1PST 12-V DC relay reed
1 Transformer, 1200 Ω ct/8 Ω
1 100-kΩ thermistor
1 VT912 photocell

INSTRUMENTATION AND BIOMEDICAL ELECTRONICS

Instrumentation is a broad title covering applications in such fields as mechanical engineering, electrical engineering, process control, fluid power, and production control. Both analog and digital problems are encountered within instrumentation. Since there are many laboratory manuals on digital instrumentation circuitry, this volume addresses primarily analog circuits.

This course is structured to stand alone; however, it could also serve as an addendum to the basic course covering the study of amplifiers, filters, and oscillators. While some analog computer circuits are included, the main emphasis is on the use of amplifiers, oscillators, timers, and transducer detectors in general instrumentation.

The circuits presented are only the tip of the iceberg. The same components, with possibly a few additions, can be used for variations of the circuits provided or in the study of many other types of circuit. Additional circuits are obtainable from data manuals listed in the bibliography. A set of these data manuals, which are nominal in cost, should be available for both student and instructor use.

In circuit drawings and descriptions, integrated circuit devices are given numbers such as MC3403, LM556, and so on. The specific code letter designations of the various manufacturers have been omitted. They do appear, however, on the technical data sheets found in the appendix.

A special phase of instrumentation, referred to herein as *biomedical electronics,* is also a very broad field covering more than 300 different types of instruments. Each instrument incorporates a variety of circuits, the study of which would require 2 years of full-time schooling. This volume is intended to familiarize you with some circuits common to biomedical instruments.

CONCLUSION

This course is designed to provide:

1. Broad coverage in the use and application of linear ICs
2. A study of circuits, parameters, and subsystems
3. A basic system of study which provides for creativeness and flexibility
4. A selection of topics which could be related to specific fields of interest
5. Coverage of standard types of circuits which could be tailored for special requirements
6. A high degree of learning with a minimum investment of time
7. Laboratory study which does not require special assembled parts
8. A study not written in "cookbook" fashion, but rather giving you the opportunity to work out required information
9. A study utilizing the latest techniques of IC design
10. Comprehensive study for students of electronics in technical colleges, vocational centers, government, military training centers, and industry

This course is challenging and interesting, and most importantly, it was enjoyable to prepare. Have a good time and enjoy your learning experience.

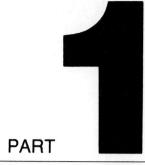

PART **1**

Amplifier
Circuits

1 NONINVERTING FOLLOWER AMPLIFIERS

OBJECTIVES

Upon completion of this experiment, construction of circuitry, testing, and evaluation of data, you will be able to:

1. *Use IC operational amplifiers as noninverting, high-gain amplifiers and as unity amplifiers*
2. *Calculate circuit component values*
3. *Compute and measure stage gain and the high-frequency roll-off points on the frequency response curve*
4. *Design operational amplifier circuits to meet specific requirements*

BACKGROUND DISCUSSION

The follower amplifier preserves the sign of the input signal. Essentially, the output V_{out} is equal to twice the input V_{in}. The output signal feedback to the negative input acts as degenerative feedback over a wide frequency range. The circuit shown in Fig. 1-1 can be used to isolate a signal source from the circuit being driven without changing the sign, phase, or amplitude of the signal.

If the feedback resistor R_2 were connected to the inverting $(-)$ input and the signal fed to the inverting $(-)$ input through R_1, the amplifier would invert the signal. The ratio of R_2/R_1 determines the voltage gain of the amplifier. If they are equal, the gain is essentially 2. If they are equal and R_4 is changed to equal R_3, the gain of the amplifier is unity. This type of amplifier might be called a *unity-gain* amplifier or follower.

EQUATIONS

$$\text{Gain } G = \frac{V_{out}}{V_{in}} \qquad (1.1)$$

$$V_{out} = V_{in} \left(1 + \frac{R_2}{R_1}\right)$$

$$\text{Where } R_2 = R_1 \text{ and } V_{out} = 2V_{in} \qquad (1.2)$$

$$\text{Gain (dB)} = 20 \log \frac{V_{out}}{V_{in}} \qquad (1.3)$$

MATERIALS REQUIRED

ACTIVE DEVICES:
  1 MC 3403
RESISTORS, 5 percent, ¼ W:
  1 1 kΩ
  3 22 kΩ
  2 100 kΩ
CAPACITORS, disc, 20 percent, 25 V
  1 0.001 μF
MISCELLANEOUS:
  1 IC socket, 14-pin
TEST INSTRUMENTS:
  Oscilloscope, dual-trace, 5-in
  Function generator, 10 Hz to 1 MHz
  Digital multimeter
  Power supply, ±15 V, 50 mA

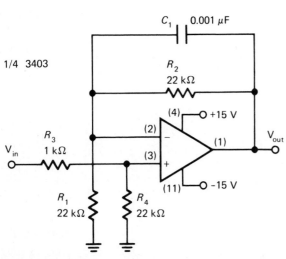

Fig. 1-1. **Noninverting amplifier**

NOTE: Use small signal levels for V_{in} to avoid saturating the amplifier. A small capacitor C_1, perhaps 0.001 μF, is connected across R_2 to stabilize the amplifier's operation and to determine its frequency response.

1. Construct the circuit shown in Fig. 1-1. Apply a small sine-wave input signal (about 5 mV peak to peak).

2. Confirm that the output-input signal ratio is approximately 2.

3. Connect the amplifier's output to the horizontal input of the oscilloscope. (See Fig. 1-2 for method of measurement.)

4. Change R_1 and R_2 to 100 kΩ each. How does this affect the gain and phase shift?

5. By changing the value of C_1, set the amplifier's high-frequency roll-off to 3 dB down at 12 kHz; i.e., make V_{out} at 12 kHz equal to 0.7 times V_{out} at the midrange.

6. Rearrange the circuit components to make the design a follower amplifier with signal inversion.

7. Check the inverter amplifier's phase shift and its gain at 1 kHz.

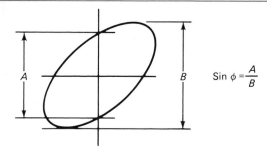

Fig. 1-2. **Measuring the phase-shift of an amplifier**

$$\text{Sin } \phi = \frac{A}{B}$$

FOR FURTHER RESEARCH

8. Design a two-amplifier system in which both amplifiers have the same input signal but the outputs are out of phase 180° and the output signal voltages are of equal amplitude. The high-frequency roll-off point of both amplifiers should be 3 dB down at 3 kHz. Compute the gain in decibels of each amplifier.

SELF-TEST

Test your knowledge of the subject by answering the following questions.

1. When you use a linear IC as a noninverting amplifier, the signal is fed into the _____ input.

2. In a noninverting amplifier, if the feedback resistor R_2 equals 100 kΩ and the resistance from the inverting input ($-$) to ground R_1 equals 1 kΩ, the stage gain is _____.

3. If $R_2 = R_1 = 10$ kΩ and $V_{in} = 1$ V, $V_{out} = $ _____.

4. If $R_2 = R_1 = 100$ kΩ and $R_3 = R_4 = 10$ kΩ, the voltage gain of the amplifier is _____.

5. If a positive-going pulse is fed into the noninverting input of the circuit in Fig. 1-1, the output pulse will be _____-going.

SELF-TEST ANSWERS
1. Noninverting ($+$)
2. 101
3. 2 V
4. Unity (1)
5. Positive

2 HIGH-GAIN INVERTING VOLTAGE AMPLIFIERS

OBJECTIVES

Upon completion of this experiment, construction of circuitry, testing, and evaluation of data, you will be able to:

1. *Use IC operational amplifiers as high-gain inverting amplifiers*
2. *Compute and measure stage gain and input resistance R_{in}*
3. *Determine an amplifier's bandwidth*
4. *Design voltage amplifiers to meet specific requirements*

BACKGROUND DISCUSSION

The operational amplifier, when connected into the circuit arrangement shown in Fig. 2-1, performs as an inverting amplifier whose gain is determined by the ratio of R_2 to R_1 (provided the gain of the IC amplifier is high). A small capacitor, its value depending on the frequency of operation desired, is placed across the feedback resistor R_2 to improve the amplifier's stability and to prevent oscillation. Capacitor C_2 may be required at low input signal levels to remove input noise; it is used also to limit the high-frequency response. Without this capacitor the frequency response will depend on the bandwidth of the chips amplifier and C_1. If the audio generator used for performing the tests has a DC component in its output, a large isolating capacitor, C_3, should be inserted at the amplifier input.

EQUATIONS

$$R_3 = \frac{R_1 R_2}{R_1 + R_2} \tag{2.1}$$

$$V_{out} \approx V_{in}\,\frac{R_2}{R_1} \tag{2.2}$$

$$\text{Gain (dB)} = 20 \log \frac{V_{out}}{V_{in}} \tag{2.3}$$

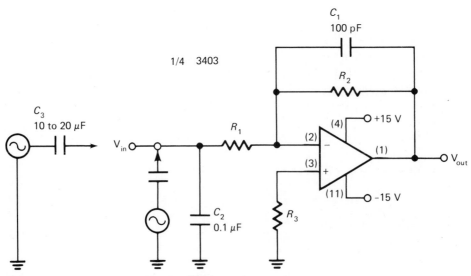

Fig. 2-1. **Phase-inverting voltage amplifier**

MATERIALS REQUIRED

ACTIVE DEVICES:
  1 MC3403
RESISTORS, 5 percent, ¼ W:
  Assortment of resistors, 100 Ω to 1 MΩ
CAPACITORS, disc, Mylar, electrolytic, 25 V:
  Assortment of capacitors, 100 pF to 0.1 μF,
  10 percent

MISCELLANEOUS COMPONENTS:
  1 IC socket, 14-pin
TEST INSTRUMENTS:
  Oscilloscope, dual-trace, 5-in
  Function generator, 10 Hz to 1 MHz
  Digital multimeter
  Power supply, $\pm$15 V, 50 mA

TESTS AND MEASUREMENTS

1. Calculate R_3 for gains of 1 to 5000 as shown in Table 2-1.

2. Validate the gains of 1 to 1000 for the resistor values listed.

3. Compute the gain in decibels for the validated gain measurements.

4. Construct the circuit shown in Fig. 2-1. Confirm the bandwidth (BW) for the gain of 1000 by measuring the 3-dB point of the high-frequency roll-off.

5. Confirm R_{in} for the gain of 100 by connecting in series a variable or decade resistor between the generator and the amplifier circuit. Measure the voltage across the series resistor and make it equal to the amplifier input signal voltage. The series resistor then equals the amplifier's input R_{in}. An alternate method is to measure the output voltage V_{out} with 0 series resistor and then increase the value of the series resistor until V_{out} is one-half its original value.

6. Change the value of C_3 so that the low-frequency 3-dB roll-off point is 10 Hz. Has your high-frequency roll-off changed? What is the bandwidth of this circuit?

7. Determine the values of R_2 and R_1 for a voltage gain of 5000 at 1 kHz.

TABLE 2-1

GAIN	R_{in}	R_1,kΩ	R_2,kΩ	BW	R_3	Gain, measured	Gain, dB
1		10	10	1 MHz			
10		1	10	100 kHz			
100		1	100	10 kHz			
1000		1	1000	1 kHz			
5000							

8. What is the purpose of C_1? How does C_1 affect the bandwidth?

FOR FURTHER RESEARCH

9. The MC3403 is one of several chips provided. Design your own amplifier, selecting another IC unit. Compute circuit component values and construct and test the circuit. Write a brief report on your findings.

10. Design a three-stage amplifier using the MC3403. The output should be inverted, overall gain equal to 100,000, and bandwidth set at 10 Hz to 3 kHz. Time permitting, test and evaluate the design.

SELF-TEST

1. When you use a linear IC as an inverter, the signal is fed into the _____ input.

2. Refer to Fig. 2-1. If $R_3 \approx 1$ kΩ, $R_2 = 20$kΩ, and $R_1 = 1$ kΩ, the stage gain is

_____ .

3. From the data provided in the Appendix, determine the typical input impedance for an MC3403.

4. Making the input coupling capacitor smaller will limit the _____-frequency roll-off.

5. The feedback capacitor limits the _____-frequency roll-off.

SELF-TEST ANSWERS

1. Inverting ($-$)
2. 20
3. 1 MΩ
4. Low
5. High

3 HIGH-GAIN NONINVERTING VOLTAGE AMPLIFIERS

OBJECTIVES

Upon completion of this experiment, construction of circuitry, testing, and evaluation of data, you will be able to:

1. *Design, construct, test, and evaluate high-gain operational amplifiers*
2. *Determine the output impedance of an operational amplifier*
3. *Determine the stage gain of an operational amplifier*

BACKGROUND DISCUSSION

This experiment is similar to Experiments 1 and 2. In this experiment, noninverting amplifiers will be evaluated and the output impedance of typical amplifiers will be measured. One specific circuit is presented, and other designs are required.

In this amplifier, as well as others you will study, a capacitor is placed across the feedback resistor in order to provide stability by limiting the amplifier's bandwidth.

The amplifier to be studied is one section of an MC3403 quad low-power operational amplifier. Its characteristics are similar to many operational amplifiers, namely, high gain, high input resistance, low input current, and low output impedance. The four sections are the same, and any one section can be used.

EQUATIONS

$$R_3 = \frac{R_1 R_2}{R_1 + R_2} \qquad (3.1)$$

$$V_{out} = V_{in} \frac{R_2}{R_1} \qquad (3.2)$$

$$\text{Gain (dB)} = 20 \log \frac{V_{out}}{V_{in}} \qquad (3.3)$$

MATERIALS REQUIRED

ACTIVE DEVICES:
    1 MC3403
RESISTORS, 5 percent, ¼ W:
    Assortment of resistors, 1 kΩ to 100 kΩ
CAPACITORS, disc, Mylar, electrolytic, 20 percent, 25 V:
    1 100 pF
    1 10 μF
MISCELLANEOUS COMPONENTS:
    1 IC socket, 14-pin
TEST INSTRUMENTS:
    Oscilloscope, dual-trace, 5 in
    Function generator, 10 Hz to 1 MHz
    Digital multimeter
    Power supply, ± 15 V, 50 mA

TESTS AND MEASUREMENTS

1. Referring to Table 3-1 and Fig. 3-1, determine R_3 for gains of 10 to 1000. Use 100 Hz on all gain measurements.
2. Construct and test the circuit shown in Fig. 3-1 and validate the circuit gain for 1000.
3. Compute the decibel gain for step 2.
4. Validate the BW for a gain of 100.
5. Determine component values for a gain of 3000 at 100 Hz.

Table 3-1

Gain	R_1,Ω	R_2*,kΩ	BW	R_{in},MΩ	R_3	R_{out}	Gain, dB
10	1	0.9	100 kHz	400			
100	100	9.9	10 kHz	200			
1000	100	99.9	1.0 Hz	80			
3000							

*Use 1-, 10-, and 100-kΩ resistors. Measure the resistance value for each resistor used to obtain closest value.

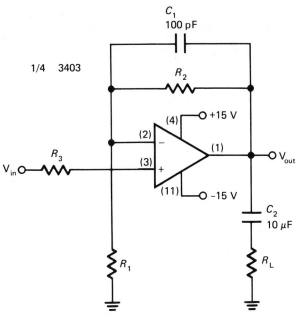

Fig. 3-1. **Noninverting high-gain amplifier**

6. With a gain of 100 and a signal source of 100 Hz, load the output circuit (see Fig. 3-1) with R_L and C_2. Determine what load-resistor value on the output reduces V_{out} by 50 percent. At this point the resistor $R_L = R_{out}$ (output resistance). Start with V_{out} equal to about 10 V (p-p).

7. What is the largest peak-to-peak input voltage that can be used without overloading the amplifier when the gain is set to 10, 1000, and 3000?

FOR FURTHER RESEARCH

8. Try designing a high-gain amplifier using an LM3900. Your amplifier should provide:
a. Gain of 10,000
b. BW of 500 Hz
c. Single-ended input and dual outputs, with one being inverted
d. Gain control

SELF-TEST

1. An amplifier has an output signal voltage of 10 V when fed with an input of 1 V. What is the stage gain in decibels?
2. What is the bandwidth of a 3403 chip?
3. Would the 3403 or any linear IC have a higher gain at 1 MHz than at 100 Hz?
4. What limits the gain of a linear IC?
5. As the gain of the amplifier is increased, the input signal voltage must be_____.

SELF-TEST ANSWERS
1. 20 dB
2. 1 MHz
3. No
4. Gain-bandwidth product
5. Decreased

EXPERIMENT 4 AC-COUPLED LOW-FREQUENCY AMPLIFIERS

OBJECTIVES

Upon completion of this experiment, construction of circuitry, testing, and evaluation of data, you will be able to:

1. *Determine the value of coupling capacitors used to cascade circuits to provide for AC coupled low-frequency amplifiers*
2. *Compute and measure the effects of using improper capacitor values for coupling circuits*
3. *Apply the same methods of measurement to circuits operating at higher frequencies*

BACKGROUND DISCUSSION

The coupling capacitor between two cascaded circuits can cause both attenuation and phase shift of the signal. At lower frequencies the problem is quite severe and can cause a loss in signal, distortion, and oscillation.

Operational amplifiers are ideal at low frequencies; however, the coupling of such amplifiers in order to handle AC signals at low frequencies can be a problem. In instrumentation, and especially biomedical instrumentation, the frequencies can get down to 0.1 Hz.

The capacitive reactance (X_C) of coupling capacitors affects the low-frequency coupling and presents problems in circuit designing.

In this experiment you will evaluate the effects of coupling and bypass capacitors on circuit design.

EQUATIONS

$$X_C = \frac{1}{6.28fC} \qquad (4.1)$$

Set $X_C = 0.05$ (5%) $R_1 = R_i$

$$X_C = 0.05R_1 \quad \text{provides rolloff} \qquad (4.2)$$

$$\text{Attenuation (dB)} = -20 \log \frac{V_{out}}{V_{in}} \qquad (4.3)$$

MATERIALS REQUIRED

ACTIVE DEVICES:
  1 MC3403
RESISTORS, 5 percent, ¼ W:
  2 1 kΩ
  1 100 kΩ
CAPACITORS, disc, Mylar, electrolytic, 20%, 25 V:
  1 100 pF
  1 10 µF, electrolytic
MISCELLANEOUS COMPONENTS:
  1 IC socket, 14-pin
TEST INSTRUMENTS:
  Oscilloscope, dual-trace, 5-in
  Function generator, 10 Hz to 1 MHz
  Digital multimeter
  Power supply, ±15 V, 50 mA

TESTS AND MEASUREMENTS

Gain

1. Construct the circuit shown in Fig. 4-1.
2. If your laboratory function generator goes down to 10 Hz, this should be the lowest frequency tested. If the generator goes only down to 20 Hz, then use this low-end frequency for testing. Feed your signal, at the lowest frequency, through a 10-µF capacitor and measure the voltage level, peak to peak, at points A and B. What percentage drop in voltage takes place at point B compared with A? From Eq. (4.3) compute the decibels of attenuation this capacitor loss represents.
3. What value of capacitor is required to limit the loss to about 1 dB?
4. If $X_C = 1000\ \Omega$, the gain of the amplifier is reduced by 50 percent. Why?

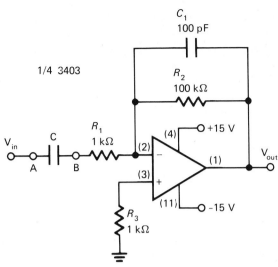

Fig. 4-1. **AC-coupled amplifier**

Phase Shift

5. Connect the vertical input of the oscilloscope to point A and the horizontal input amplifier (no sweep) to point B. Test a 1-μF capacitor, as well as smaller and larger values, to see the effect of the coupling capacitor on phase shift. How much shift occurs at 10 Hz, 100 Hz, and 1 kHz?

The elliptical pattern is a measure of the phase shift present. (Refer to Experiment 1 for previous measurements of phase shift or ask your instructor for assistance in making the measurement).

6. At 10 or 20 Hz, how much phase shift do a 10- and a 100-μF capacitor cause?

7. Assume that resistor R_3 has to be bypassed. What size capacitor is required if the circuit is to work down to 1 Hz?

FOR FURTHER RESEARCH

8. While phase shifting may be undesirable in some circuits, it is desirable in oscillators and filters. In the twin-T oscillator, RC circuits are designed so that the phase-shifted output signal, when fed back to the input of the amplifier, will cause the amplifier to oscillate.

Design a low-frequency amplifier with an overall gain of 100,000 and with a low-frequency response to 0.5 Hz. The upper roll-off point should be 100 Hz. Use the MC3403 for your design.

SELF-TEST

1. What is the capacitive reactance of a 0.01-μF capacitor when used in a circuit operating at 10 Hz?

2. An amplifier circuit is operating between 100 Hz and 10 kHz. The input resistor is 10 kΩ. What minimum size of coupling capacitor is recommended?

3. From your laboratory experiences or from technical data sheets, would you estimate the output impedance of the MC3403 to be: *(a)* 300 to 800 Ω, *(b)* 20 to 100 Ω, *(c)* 500 to 1000 Ω, *(d)* above 1000 Ω?

4. What is (are) the advantage(s) of using a 10-μF tantalum capacitor for coupling rather than a 10-μF electrolytic capacitor?

5. Is polarity of the coupling capacitor a factor when you connect an electrolytic between two stages?

SELF-TEST ANSWERS

1. 1.59 MΩ
2. 3 μF (approximate)
3. *b*
4. Less leakage current
5. Yes, positive terminal goes to the positive voltage

5 HIGH-INPUT IMPEDANCE AMPLIFIERS

OBJECTIVES

Upon completion of this experiment, construction of circuitry, testing, and evaluation of data, you will be able to:

1. *Measure the input impedance of an operational amplifier*
2. *Change component values which affect the amplifier's input impedance*
3. *Determine the amplifier's bandwidth and determine its response by selecting feedback loop components*

BACKGROUND DISCUSSION

High–input-impedance amplifiers are useful for the design of filters and bridge circuits, for input transducers, and for making measurements on high-resistance sources. For example, the human body has a skin resistance of from 50,000 Ω to nearly 1 MΩ. If a low–input-resistance amplifier were used for making measurements, the amplifier would appear as a shunting load, and hence the measurements being made would not be correct.

In this experiment an amplifier uses a feedback loop to increase the input impedance so that the amplifier's input is in the 100-MΩ region. The amplifier gain is at or near unity and is noninverting. The output impedance is low and hence good for driving a meter.

MATERIALS REQUIRED

ACTIVE DEVICES:
  1 MC3403
RESISTORS, 5 percent, ¼ W:
  Assortment of resistors, 1 kΩ to 1 MΩ
CAPACITORS, disc, Mylar, electrolytic, 20%, 25 V:
  Assortment of capacitors, 0.001 to 20 μF
MISCELLANEOUS COMPONENTS:
  1 IC socket, 14-pin
TEST INSTRUMENTS:
  Oscilloscope, dual-trace, 5 in
  Function generator, 10 Hz to 1 MHz
  Digital multimeter
  Power supply, $\pm$15 V, 50 mA

TESTS AND MEASUREMENTS

1. Construct the circuit in Fig. 5-1 using component values shown. Determine the amplifier's input resistance by connecting resistors in series with the input (shown as R_x). Feed in a signal of 100 Hz and adjust the generator so that V_{out} is 10 V when $R_x = 0$. Increase the value of R_x until $V_{out} = 5$ Vs. At this point the voltage drop V_1 across R_x is equal to the amplifier's input voltage V_2, and so the amplifier input resistance R_{in} equals R_x. Since the input resistance is quite high, R_x will be made up of 20-, 10-, and 5-MΩ resistors.

2. Determine what effect C_2 has on input resistance by using a 100 Hz signal source and by reducing C_2 first to a 0.1-μF and then a 0.05-μF capacitor. The X_C of capacitor C_2 acts as a feedback resistor. As the fre-

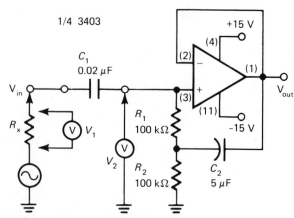

Fig. 5-1. **High–input-impedance amplifier**

quency goes down, X_C increases; hence the feedback is reduced. Record R_x for each value of C_2.

3. Compute the value of X_C at 10 Hz for a 0.05-, 0.1-, and 5-μF capacitor. Since the feedback voltage is developed across R_f, what percentage of the output voltage is fed back at 100 Hz when $C_2 = 5 \ \mu$F?

4. Determine R_{in} when $C_2 = 10 \ \mu$F.

FOR FURTHER RESEARCH

5. Design an amplifier which has an input impedance of 50 MΩ, a gain of 10,000, a bandwidth of 1 kHz, and a low-frequency response of 1 Hz. Use several sections of a 3403, 3900, or such other quad operational amplifier as you desire.

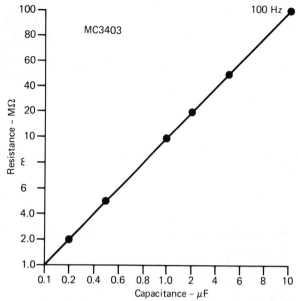

Fig. 5-2. **Feedback capacitor, value versus input resistance**

SELF-TEST

1. If a low-resistance voltmeter is used to measure the voltage drop across a 10-MΩ resistor, what will be the effect?

2. A voltage-follower circuit was used in the experiment. What is the gain of such a circuit?

3. Is the output impedance of a voltage-follower circuit increased when feedback is provided?

4. Is the effective input impedance of the experiment circuit greater or less than $R_1 + R_2$?

5. If an amplifier is to operate down to 10 Hz, does the required input coupling capacitor get smaller or larger as the input impedance is made larger?

SELF-TEST ANSWERS

1. Meter will load the circuit and incorrect reading will be obtained.

2. Unity

3. No

4. Greater

5. Smaller

6 HIGH-GAIN QUAD AMPLIFIERS

EXPERIMENT

OBJECTIVES

Upon completion of this experiment, construction of circuitry, testing, and evaluation of data, you will be able to:

1. *Select one or more quad IC chips to be used for amplifier applications*
2. *Design, construct, and test amplifiers as required to meet design constraints*
3. *Design amplifiers to meet desired bandwidth requirements*

BACKGROUND DISCUSSION

In the development of linear ICs (operational amplifiers), designs have progressed from one amplifier per chip, as in the 741 or 709, to dual amplifiers, such as the 747, to quad amplifiers. A number of different types of quads are available. Some have high gain and low output impedance, and others have a high output impedance. Some amplifiers have a gain of unity at 1 MHz, and others go to 2.5 MHz and higher. Some amplifiers are better-suited to be used as comparators; others make good oscillators. There are many to choose from, and all are economical.

In this experiment the LM324 has been selected to illustrate a type of IC which, like the LM3900, requires additional biasing of one input for proper operation.

In most amplifiers the gain of a stage is determined by the ratio of the feedback resistor R_f to the series input resistor R_{in}. This assumes that the amplification A_0 of the amplifier is high, which it is in most ICs.

In the circuit of Fig. 6-1, the noninverting input (pin 5) is biased by two resistors, R_3 and R_4. Later you will refer to the technical notes in the Appendix for the LM3900, a different but similar quad, and you will test this amplifier with variations in biasing. You should also make a comparison between the internal wiring and components used in the 324 and those used in the 3403.

The ICs designated by number in this and other experiments may be interchangeable with others in a series. For example, Motorola lists the 3403 as MC3503L, or MC3403P or L. The 3503 is the same as the 3403 except that the temperature range of operation is broader. The L or P indicates whether the case is ceramic or plastic. Basically, the IC is the same.

In this experiment the 324 is used as a phase-inverter amplifier whose gain you will both compute and measure.

EQUATIONS

$$\text{Stage gain} = \frac{R_f}{R_{in}} \qquad (6.1)$$

$$\text{Gain (dB)} = 20 \log \frac{V_{out}}{V_{in}} \qquad (6.2)$$

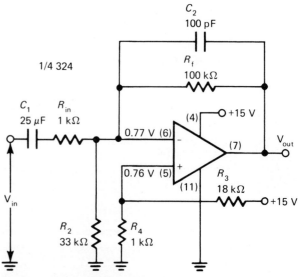

Fig. 6-1. **Phase inverter using one-fourth of a quad amplifier**

MATERIALS REQUIRED

ACTIVE DEVICES:
   1 LM324
   1 LM3900
   1 MC3403

RESISTORS, 5 percent, ¼ W:
   2 1 kΩ
   1 18 kΩ
   1 33 kΩ
   1 100 kΩ

CAPACITORS, 20 percent, 25 V:
   1 100 pF disc
   1 25 μF electrolytic

MISCELLANEOUS COMPONENTS:
   1 IC socket, 14-pin

TEST INSTRUMENTS:
   Oscilloscope, dual-trace, 5-in
   Function generator, 10 Hz to 1 MHz
   Digital multimeter
   Power supply, $\pm$15 V, 50 mA

TESTS AND MEASUREMENTS

During your laboratory exercises you will first evaluate one amplifier on the LM324, then you will conduct similar tests on an MC3403 and on an LM3900. The LM3900 makes use of what is known as a Norton amplifier.

1. Construct the circuit in Fig. 6-1 using component values as shown. Record your static-input voltages (voltages with no signal).

2. Measure the stage gain at 100 Hz using a 50-mV p-p input signal (state gain also in decibels). What is the maximum driving signal before saturation or cutoff occurs? Record the maximum undistorted output voltage V_{out}.

3. Determine the upper-end roll-off point using capacitor C_2 as shown.

4. Repeat steps 2 and 3 using a square-wave signal $V_{in} = 50$ mV with leading edge of 1 ms. At what frequency does the square wave start to look like a sine wave? Which edge, leading or trailing, of the square wave represents high-frequency components?

5. Repeat these tests using the 3900. Use data in the Appendix as necessary. Determine which IC appears to be easier to work with for this simple amplifier arrangement—the 324, 3900, or 3403 of Experiment 4.

6. On the last amplifier tested (the 3900) try changing the feedback resistor from a fixed 100-kΩ resistor to a 100-kΩ potentiometer. Use the center terminal (wiper) and one end terminal.

7. With the full 100-kΩ potentiometer resistance, the amplifier is the same as previously tested; however, by varying the resistance ratio, you vary the gain of the amplifier ($G = R_f/R_{in}$). This circuit provides an arrangement whereby you control the signal level being processed by controlling stage gain rather than by controlling the input signal level to the amplifier. Adjust the amplifier gain to unity and measure the value of R_f. Does $R_f = R_{in}$?

FOR FURTHER RESEARCH

8. Design an AC-coupled amplifier using three units of the LM3900 to provide a gain of 10,000. Use the fourth amplifier as a buffer amplifier with high input impedance and unity gain. Your frequency response should be 100 Hz. Provide a circuit with static voltages, a frequency response curve, and gain calculations in decibels. Time permitting, construct the amplifier and verify your design.

SELF-TEST

   1. The large-scale voltage gain of an LM324 is_____, compared with_____ for a 3403.

   2. *Slew rate* is defined as the change in_____over a period of_____.

   3. The LM3900 has an output resistance of_____. The output resistance of the 3403 is_____.

   4. The common mode rejection ratio (CMRR) of an LM324 is_____, while that of the 3403 is_____.

   5. Which of the three chips (324, 3403, 3900) has the best power-supply rejection ratio?

SELF-TEST ANSWERS

   1. 100; 200   **4.** 70; 90
   2. Volts; 1 μs   **5.** The 324 is best
   3. 8 kΩ, 75 Ω   (324-100, 3403-30, 3900-70)

EXPERIMENT 7 LOW-FREQUENCY BASS-BOOST AMPLIFIERS

OBJECTIVES

Upon completion of this experiment, construction of circuitry, testing, and evaluation of data, you will be able to:

1. *Use operational amplifiers for the design of high-gain, low-frequency amplification systems*
2. *Test and evaluate bass-boost circuitry used in an audio amplifier for increasing low-frequency response*
3. *Incorporate high-frequency roll-off circuits in audio amplifiers*

BACKGROUND DISCUSSION

Low-frequency amplifiers have application in the entertainment field, instrumentation, and biomedical instrumentation. While the audio listening range may be limited on the low end to 20 to 30 Hz, there are lower-frequency sounds which can be recorded and evaluated. In this experiment emphasis is given to the use of very-low-frequency amplifiers, boosting the low frequencies, and using feedback gain control.

In the biomedical field, phonocardiography is the recording of heart sounds. While most heart sounds are in the range of 25 to 2000 Hz, some pressure sounds go to under 1 Hz. The following is a listing of some heart sound frequencies:

1. Low- and high-pitch heart murmurs, under 400 Hz
2. Breathing, 240 to 660 Hz
3. Lowest-frequency heart sound, 5 to 10 Hz
4. Other sounds, 250 to 2000 Hz

Special microphones, filters, and amplifiers are required for such applications. Filters are used to attenuate specified frequency ranges so that the listener can concentrate on sounds in the desired frequency range.

Audio amplifiers with limited frequency response are also used in the communications field. Usually 300 to 3000 Hz is used for speech communications. The elimination of the highs and lows of the audio amplifier reduces the difficulty in modulation and the filtering of RF sideband radiation.

Amplifier gain and attenuation are usually rated in terms of decibels. The term *decibel* refers to a logarithmic change in the intensity of sound. When gain in decibels is plotted against frequency, a frequency-response curve is produced, which graphically illustrates an amplifier's performance at varying frequencies. Filters often have a roll-off or filter slope of 12 dB per octave. The term "-12 dB" refers to a reduction in intensity to 0.251 times the midband intensity. An octave is a musical term which refers to a change in frequency or pitch by a factor of 2. A $12-$dB roll-off of an amplifier at 2000 Hz means the final intensity from the amplifier will be reduced by 0.251 times the 1000 Hz intensity.

The circuit you will study in this experiment is only a preamplifier. To this can be added a power amplifier for driving a loudspeaker, modulator, or servo-control system. The IC used here is not the best choice for the application. A low-noise amplifier such as the CA3048 or CA3052 or the equivalent is recommended where low-level sounds are to be recorded. However, the 3403 will demonstrate all of the necessary points to be learned.

The circuit in Fig. 7-1 consists of four amplifiers, one using a single transistor. The transistor amplifier is used to provide additional bass boost. Since the interest is in low-frequency amplification, treble-boost circuitry has been omitted. Gain is provided by feedback control on the second amplifier. In feedback control the gain of the amplifier's entire output is fed back to the inverted input. The gain of the second amplifier is determined by the ratio of the gain-control resistance R_8 to the input resistance R_7. High frequencies are passed by C_3, but low frequencies are shunted to the bass-boost

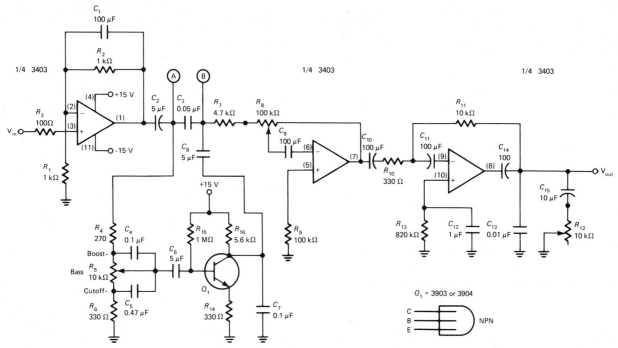

Fig. 7-1. **Low-frequency bass-boost amplifier**

control, amplified, and reintroduced at point B along with the high frequencies. C_{15} and R_{12} provide a load to test the circuit.

While the circuit provides for one amplifier, two such amplifiers would provide for stereo. While the 3403 is used in the project, the CA3052 is a quad amplifier better suited for this application.

EQUATIONS

$$\text{Gain } G_2 = \frac{R_f}{R_{in}} = \frac{R_8}{R_7} = \frac{R_{11}}{R_{10}} \quad (7.1)$$

$$\text{Gain (dB)} = 20 \log \frac{V_{out}}{V_{in}} \quad (7.2)$$

MATERIALS REQUIRED

ACTIVE DEVICES:
1 LM3403
1 2N3904 transistor

RESISTORS, 5 percent, ¼ W:

1 100 Ω	1 10 kΩ
1 270 Ω	1 100 kΩ
3 330 Ω	1 820 kΩ
2 1000 Ω	1 1 MΩ
1 4.7 kΩ	1 5.6 kΩ

2 10 kΩ potentiometer, linear, ½ W
1 100 kΩ potentiometer, linear, ½ W

CAPACITORS, disc, Mylar, electrolytic, 20 percent, 25 V:

1 100 pF	1 1.0 μF
1 0.01 μF	3 5 μF
1 0.05 μF	1 10 μF
2 0.1 μF	4 100 μF
1 0.47 μF	

MISCELLANEOUS COMPONENTS:
IC socket, 14 pin

TEST INSTRUMENTS:
Oscilloscope, dual-trace, 5 in
Function generator, 10 Hz to 1 MHz
Digital multimeter
Power supply, ±15 V, 50 mA

TESTS AND MEASUREMENTS

1. Construct the circuit shown in Fig. 7-1 and test the overall operation by feeding in a 50- to 100-Hz signal. Look at V_{out} on an oscilloscope. Try adjusting the gain control and bass control and adjust the input signal so that overloading does not take place. If the circuit does not function properly, troubleshoot each amplifier, starting with the first stage.

2. Check the amplifier's overall voltage gain and gain in decibels. Determine the decibel gain separately for each stage. Use a 100-Hz signal and set the bass control to midrange and the high-frequency control to maximum.

3. Repeat the gain measurements with the bass control first at maximum and again at minimum.

4. How much added bass boost is provided by the circuitry of Q_1? Try removing the bass-boost amplifier from the circuit by removing capacitor C_8 and connecting the signal output of C_6 (5 μF) directly to point B.

5. Record all operating voltages (no signal applied).

6. What is the amplifier's lowest manageable frequency?

7. What is the highest input signal voltage acceptable without output distortion?

FOR FURTHER RESEARCH

8. Try connecting your amplifier to a loudspeaker.

SELF-TEST

Refer to the circuit in Fig. 7-1.

1. The calculated gain of the first amplifier is _____.

2. The maximum gain of the second IC amplifier is_____.

3. Capacitor C_3 passes the _____frequencies, while the _____ frequencies are amplified by Q_1 and passed through C_8.

4. Does the circuit have treble boast?

5. A positive-going input signal results in a _____-going output signal.

SELF-TEST ANSWERS

1. 2
2. 21 (approximately)
3. High; low
4. No
5. Positive

PART REVIEW: AMPLIFIERS

1. To make a noninverting amplifier, to which input must the signal be fed?
2. Draw a circuit for a noninverting amplifier and indicate which two resistors determine the gain of the amplifier.
3. How is an amplifier's high-frequency response controlled?
4. Do operational amplifiers, such as the MC3403, have a low or high output impedance? State the range in ohms.
5. What factors determine the choice of a coupling capacitor between two amplifiers?
6. Does the coupling capacitor affect the high- or low-frequency response?
7. Draw a circuit for a high–input-resistance (50- to 100-MΩ) amplifier. As the input resistance goes up, what happens to the amplifier's gain?
8. What is the difference between a 3503 and a 3403 chip?
9. Draw three circuits showing how the gain of an amplifier can be controlled.
10. Draw a circuit showing two unity-gain amplifiers which can produce two out-of-phase signals from a single signal input.

PART **2**

Instrumentation Circuits

8 HIGH-IMPEDANCE INSTRUMENT AMPLIFIERS

OBJECTIVES

Upon completion of this experiment, construction of circuitry, testing, and evaluation of data, you will be able to:

1. *Design, test, and evaluate high-input resistance amplifiers which use integrated circuits*
2. *Evaluate operational amplifier circuits which utilize resistance multiplication*
3. *Determine the gain of high-input resistance amplifiers*

DISCUSSION

The gain of an operational amplifier is determined by the ratio of R_f to R_{in}. If the amplifier is to provide both gain and high-input resistance, the values of R_f and R_{in} become very large. In this experiment a circuit design is presented in which gain and high-input resistance is obtainable. Referring to the circuit shown in Fig. 8-1, the output of the amplifier contains a voltage divider (R_4 and R_3) with a ratio of 10:1. The amplifier has a high gain; however, unity gain feedback is provided to the input.

A disadvantage of the circuit is that the input offset voltage is increased at the output. The output-voltage offset follows the equation

$$V_{out} = (\frac{R_1 + R_2}{R_2}) A_V V_{os}$$

where V_{os} is the input offset voltage and V_{out} is the resultant output. The gain of the amplifier is determined by four resistors rather than two. Resistor tolerances thus become more of a problem. The gain of the amplifier is determined by the equation

$$G = \frac{R_2(R_3 + R_4)}{R_1 R_3}$$

where R_2 should be greater than R_1 and much greater than R_3. The value of R_1 determines the input resistance, and its value can be made larger if a smaller gain is acceptable. The value of R_4 is usually made 10 to 100 times larger than R_3. Depending on the gain and input resistance desired, the ratio of R_4 to R_3 can be altered. The amplifier is of the inverting type.

In the conventional operational amplifier, suppose that an input resistance of 2 MΩ is required, with a gain of 100. The resistors for R_{in} and R_f would be $R_{in} = $ 2 MΩ and $R_f = $ 200 MΩ. The value of R_f would be difficult to handle in practical circuits. Recall that

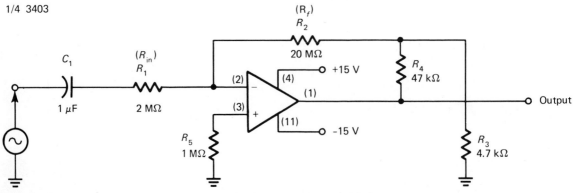

Fig. 8–1. **High-input impedance amplifier.**

$(R_4/R_3) = 10$. Suppose that $R_1 = 2\,M\Omega$, $R_2 = 20\,M\Omega$, $R_3 = 4.7\,k\Omega$, and $R_4 = 47\,k\Omega$; then

$$G = \frac{2 \times 10^7 (4.7 \times 10^3 + 47 \times 10^3)}{2 \times 10^6 \times 4.7 \times 10^3}$$

$$= \frac{1.034 \times 10^{12}}{9.4 \times 10^9} = 1.1 \times 10^2$$

$$= 110$$

Thus it can be seen that the amplifier has a high gain with $R_f = 20\,M\Omega$ rather than 200 MΩ. When it is desirable to reduce the effect of the output voltage offset, R_2 is increased in value. This change need not be made to practical circuits if the voltage offset at the output is not a problem. The amplifier is useful where high-resistance transducers are to be used and where gain is required.

EQUATIONS

$$G = \frac{R_2(R_3 + R_4)}{R_1 R_3} \qquad (8\text{-}1)$$

where: R_2 is greater than R_1
R_2 is much greater than R_3
R_4 is 10 to 100 times greater than R_3

MATERIALS REQUIRED

ACTIVE DEVICES:
  1 MC3403
RESISTORS: 5%, 1/4 W
  1 4.7 kΩ
  1 47 kΩ
  1 1 MΩ
  1 2 MΩ
  1 20 MΩ
CAPACITORS: disc, Mylar, electrolytic, 20%, 25 V
  1 1 μF
MISCELLANEOUS COMPONENTS:
  1 Socket, 14-pin
TEST INSTRUMENTS:
  Oscilloscope, dual-trace, 5-in
  Function generator, 10 Hz-to-1 MHz
  Digital multimeter
  Power supply, ±15 V, 50 mA

TESTS AND MEASUREMENTS

1. Construct the circuit shown in Fig. 8-1 using the component values indicated. Record IC pin voltages with no signal applied.

2. Measure the gain at 25 Hz using an input signal that does not overload the amplifier (about 0.04 V p-p).

3. Compute the gain using Eq. (8-1) and compare with measured value. [Substitute *measured* values of resistances in Eq. (8-1).]

4. Compute the output voltage offset.

5. Assume that output offset is not a problem and the input requirement is a resistance of 10 MΩ. If $R_2 = R_1$, $R_4 = 47\,k\Omega$, and $R_3 = 4.7\,k\Omega$, what is the gain of the amplifier? Measure all components actually used for values substituted in Eq. (8-1). Check the computed gain against the measured gain.

6. What is the maximum input signal that the amplifier in step 5 can handle at 25 Hz?

7. At what high frequency does the output drop to the 3-dB point?

SELF-TEST

Test your comprehension of the subject by answering the following questions.

1. The input resistance of the circuit in Fig. 8-1 is determined by _____.
2. Is the gain of the circuit in Fig. 8-1 greater or less than the ratio of R_2 to R_1?
3. At low signal levels, a large input resistance also increases the _____ of the amplifier.
4. The circuit in Fig. 8-1 provides phase inversion (true or false).
5. As the gain of an amplifier increases, its dynamic signal input range _____.

SELF-TEST ANSWERS
1. R_1
2. Greater
3. Noise
4. True
5. Decreases

9 DIFFERENTIAL INPUT INSTRUMENT AMPLIFIERS

OBJECTIVES

Upon completion of this experiment, testing, and evaluation of data, you will be able to:

1. *Test and troubleshoot differential amplifiers which use linear integrated circuits*

2. *Determine the common-mode rejection ratio of differential amplifiers*

3. *Determine the stage gain of differential amplifiers*

4. *Determine the bandwidth of differential amplifiers*

DISCUSSION

The differential amplifier is used when a difference voltage has to be measured in the presence of other, undesired voltages. In the medical instrument field the heart's electrical output potentials across the human chest produce voltages in the microvolt and millivolt range. Measuring such voltages across two points on the chest, in the presence of voltages produced by power-line fields (50 Hz or 60 Hz), would be a problem unless the power-line voltages could be filtered out. There are many similar applications in the instrument field where a difference voltage is to be measured and the in-phase voltage reduced.

The differential amplifier consists basically of two amplifiers whose emitter sections are controlled by a constant-current control circuit. The output can be taken from both amplifiers (twice the gain of one amplifier) or from one (gain of one amplifier only). Figure 9-1 shows the basic arrangement for a differential amplifier. If two out-of-phase signals are fed to amplifiers *A* and *B* and if their amplitudes are equal, the voltage drop across R_E (for two opposite but equal currents) will be zero, and the gain of both amplifiers will be available. If a common signal (in phase) is fed to both amplifiers, the currents from *A* and *B* will be in phase $(I_1 + I_2)$ and a voltage drop will occur across R_E. This voltage is degenerative, as is any emitter resistor pro-

vided in an amplifier, and the gain of the two amplifiers is reduced.

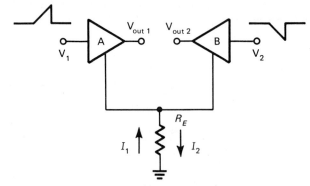

Fig. 9–1. **The concept of differential amplifiers.**

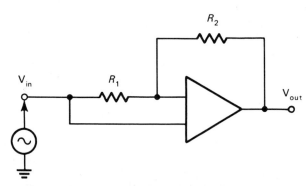

Fig. 9–2. **Method for measuring common-mode rejection (CMR).**

The CMRR defines how much attenuation will take place between output and input for an in-phase signal. Figure 9-2 shows the basic circuit arrangement for measuring the CMRR. The measurement of $V_{out} - V_{in}$ is difficult and since attenuation of the common-mode signal is desired, the common-mode rejection (CMR) provided by the amplifier is

$$\text{CMR} = 20 \log_{10} \left(- \frac{V_{out}}{V_{in}} \right)$$

expressed in decibels. The gain of the out-of-phase signal voltage is as follows:

$$A_v = -\frac{V_{out}}{V_{in}} = -V_{in} \times A + \frac{V_{out,CM}}{CMR}$$

where A is the amplification factor. If $V_{out,CM}$ (common-mode output) is very small compared to the ratio of V_{out} to V_{in}, it can almost be neglected and $A_v = -(V_{out}/V_{in})$ (the $-$ meaning the signal is inverted). If the output is taken from only one amplifier the gain becomes

$$A_V = \frac{V_{out}/V_{in}}{2}$$

In this experiment the gain and CMR are measured, and also the bandwidth (BW) response of the amplifier is limited to low-frequency applications. Two operational amplifiers (A and B) are used in a differential circuit arrangement. The third amplifier (C) has a differential input and single output.

DEFINITIONS

Common-Mode Rejection (CMR)

This is the ability of the differential amplifier to reject (i.e., produce no output as a result of) in-phase, equal-amplitude signals appearing simultaneously at the inputs. If $V_{in1} = V_{in2}$, then $V_{out} = 0$ since $V_{in1} - V_{in2} = 0$.

Common-Mode Rejection Ratio (CMRR)

This is the ratio of a differential amplifier's ability to reject common-mode (in-phase, equal-amplitude) signals appearing simultaneously at its inputs to its ability to differential (out-of-phase) signals appearing simultaneously at its inputs. Usually the ratio is expressed in the negative decibel (loss) equivalent.

In determining the CMRR the two signals (common-mode and differential) are adjusted at the input to produce the same output voltage. For example, if a 10-V common-mode signal produces an output of 0.2 V and a differential signal of 10 mV also produces an output of 0.2 V, then CMRR = (10/0.01) = (1000/1) or expressed in negative decibels,

$$20 \log_{10} \frac{V_{in,CM}}{V_{in,DIFF}} = 20 \log_{10} \frac{10}{0.01}$$
$$= 20 \log_{10} 1000$$
$$= -60 \text{ dB}$$

Differential amplifiers are rated in terms of the number of decibel attenuation to common-mode signals.

EQUATIONS

Referring to Fig. 9-3, let $R_1 = R_4$ (match values of resistors or use resistor combinations to obtain equals).

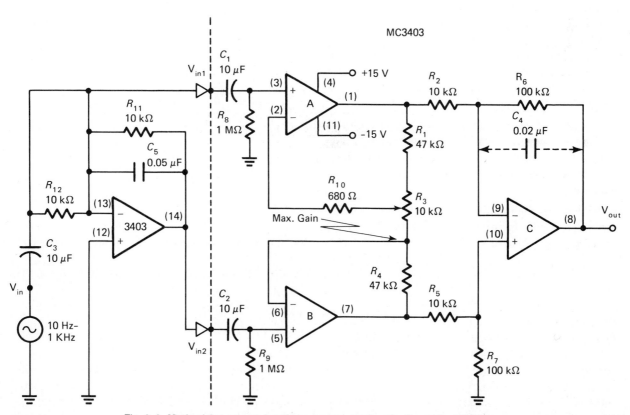

Fig. 9–3. **Method for measuring the common-mode rejection ratio (CMRR).**

$$R_2 = R_5 \text{ (mismatch reduces CMR)}$$

$$R_6 = R_7 \tag{9-1}$$

$$A_V = \frac{R_6}{R_2}\left(1 + \frac{2R_1}{R_3}\right) \tag{9-2}$$

$$\text{CMR (dB)} = 20 \log_{10} \frac{V_{\text{out}}}{V_{\text{in}}}$$

for in-phase signal $\tag{9-3}$

$$V_{\text{out}} = \frac{R_6}{R_2}\left(1 + \frac{R_1}{R_3}\right)(V_2 - V_1) \tag{9-4}$$

$$\text{CMRR} = 20 \log_{10} \frac{A_{\text{CM}}}{A_{\text{DIFF}}} \tag{9-5}$$

expressed in decibels.

MATERIALS REQUIRED

ACTIVE DEVICES:
  1 MC3403
RESISTORS: 5%, 1/4 W
  1 680 Ω
  4 10 kΩ
  2 47 kΩ
  2 100 kΩ
  2 1 MΩ
  1 10-kΩ Potentiometer
CAPACITORS: disc, Mylar, electrolytic, 20%, 25 V
  1 0.02 μF
  1 0.05 μF
  3 10 μF
MISCELLANEOUS COMPONENTS:
  1 Socket, 14-pin
TEST INSTRUMENTS:
  Oscilloscope, dual-trace, 5-in
  Function generator, 10 Hz to 1 MHz
  Digital multimeter
  Power supply, $\pm$15 V, 50 mA

TESTS AND MEASUREMENTS

CMR Measurement

1. Construct the circuit shown in Fig. 9-3 using component values as shown. Measure and record static voltages (no signal applied) with the gain control at minimum and the input of the phase splitter shorted to ground. (**NOTE:** The 680-Ω (R_{10}) resistor in series with the arm of the gain control is to prevent shorting of inputs 2 and 6 when the wiper is set to maximum gain nearest R_4.)

2. a. Connect the two inputs (pins 3 and 5) as shown in Fig. 9-4. Connect a 100-Hz, 2-V p-p common-mode signal from the audio generator to point A and measure the output voltage V_{out} (pin 8) with the gain control at maximum.

b. Now adjust the input signal so as to obtain a 0.2-V p-p output signal (gain at maximum) and record the required input voltage, V_{in}.

3. Compute the CMR using data obtained in step 2b.

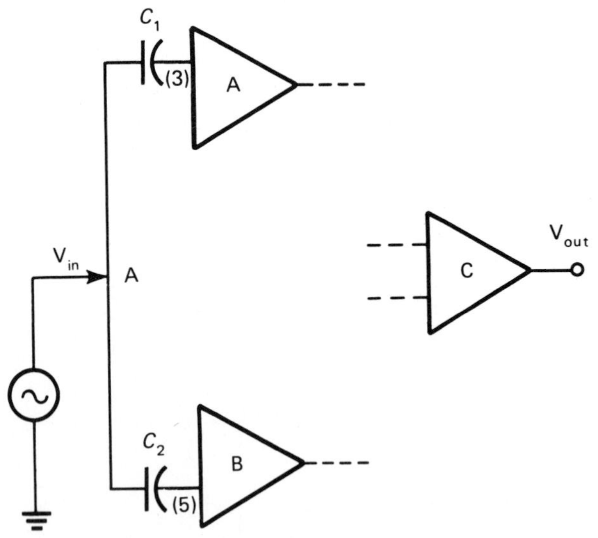

Gain Measurement

NOTE: Most function generators do not have differential outputs, so the required out-of-phase signal will be produced by the phase-splitter circuit made from the remaining operational amplifier on the chip. Some oscilloscopes have only a single input. To determine $V_{\text{in,DIFF}}$, it is necessary to measure V_{in1} and V_{in2} separately and ascertain the differential input signal algebraically:

Fig. 9–4. **Method for measuring the common-mode ratio (CMR).**

$$V_{\text{in,DIFF}} = V_{\text{in1}} - V_{\text{in2}}$$

Two methods of measuring $V_{\text{in,DIFF}}$ are common when dual-trace scopes are employed, depending on operating modes. For scopes having switch-selectable $A - B$ modes (single-trace algebraic difference of channels

A and B), the value of the differential signal appearing at the inputs is easily determined. For scopes without such a mode of operation, the two signals can be brought close together so that they just touch, and then V_{in1} is added to V_{in2}.

4. a. Configure the circuit again so that the differentiator is connected to the input of the differential amplifier. Set $V_{in,DIFF} = 10$ mV (reference is made to the "note" above) and while observing V_{out}, adjust the gain control for the maximum undistorted output. *Do not* move the gain control for the remaining parts of this step. Compute the gain at 100 Hz.

b. Now adjust $V_{in,DIFF}$ to obtain a 0.2-V p-p output. Measure and record the required $V_{in,DIFF}$.

c. Compute the CMRR in decibels using data obtained in steps 2b and 4b.

5. Referring to step 4b, compute the theoretical output voltage and compare it with the measured values.

6. What is the maximum differential signal the am-plifier can handle (set the gain control to midrange).

7. Induce roll-off of the high-frequency response by placing a 0.02-μF capacitor across R_6. Make a frequency-response test from 10 Hz to 1 kHz and determine where roll-off occurs (3-dB point).

FOR FURTHER RESEARCH

8. The differential signal to be measured in a system is 1 mV and the noise-stray pickup is 5 mV. Using your original circuit, determine how much signal and how much noise will appear at the output and compare the two values. What is the ratio of $V_{out(signal)}/V_{n\,(noise)}$?

9. As a result of brain-wave voltages, the differential signal on your head is 10 to 50 μV at frequencies under 40 Hz. How much gain should your amplifier have in order to obtain 0.5 V/cm on your oscilloscope? Design a differential amplifier circuit that would make these measurements.

SELF-TEST

Test your comprehension of the subject by answering the following questions.

1. Each amplifier section of an MC3403 is a _____ amplifier.
2. The CMRR of an MC3403 amplifier is rated at _____ dB.
3. Is the gain of amplifiers A and B in the experiment greater or less than the ratio of $2R_1$ to R_3?
4. The term *common-mode rejection ratio* relates to the ratio of a common mode to differential signal to produce the same signal output (true or false).
5. Magnetically induced voltages produce common-mode signals (true or false).

SELF-TEST ANSWERS
1. Differential
2. 90
3. Greater
4. True
5. True

10
CONSTANT-VOLTAGE REFERENCE SOURCES

OBJECTIVES

Upon completion of this experiment, construction of circuitry, testing, and evaluation of data, you will be able to:

1. *Test and evaluate voltage reference sources*
2. *Design voltage reference sources for specific requirements*
3. *Use integrated circuits in the design of voltage reference sources*

DISCUSSION

Instrumentation circuitry, such as comparators, voltage-level shifters, and bridges, may require fixed or variable voltage references. Two circuits will be constructed in this experiment, namely, a positive and a negative voltage reference source. In each circuit direct feedback from the output to the negative input is provided, and the positive input is provided with a variable biasing voltage.

The operational amplifier lends itself well to a reference source application since it has a low output resistance which is not easily loaded by external circuits.

MATERIALS REQUIRED

ACTIVE DEVICES:
  1 MC3403
RESISTORS: 5%, 1/4 W
  1 330 Ω
  1 1 kΩ
  1 10-kΩ potentiometer
MISCELLANEOUS COMPONENTS:
  1 Socket, 14-pin
TEST INSTRUMENTS:
  Oscilloscope, dual-trace, 5-in
  Function generator, 10 Hz to 1 MHz
  Digital multimeter
  Power supply, $\pm$15 V, 50 mA

TESTS AND MEASUREMENTS

1. Construct the positive voltage reference circuit shown in Fig. 10-1 and check the no-load output voltage range provided by the 10-kΩ potentiometer. Record the voltage range and voltage polarity.

2. Set the output at 6.0 V and load the output using a resistance decade box or other variable resistance load of 200 Ω to 10 kΩ. (*Suggestion:* Don't go below 200 Ω since the current range of the IC will be exceeded and the IC may be damaged.) Does the voltage remain constant under load? Plot the output voltage against the load resistance.

3. Look at the voltage output with an AC-coupled oscilloscope. Does noise or ripple appear? How much? What can you do to reduce the noise or ripple?

4. Redesign the voltage range circuitry to limit the output to 4 to 8 V.

5. Construct the negative-voltage reference circuit shown in Fig. 10-2 and perform the tests of steps 1 through 4 again.

FOR FURTHER RESEARCH

6. How much current is flowing through the IC output under the 200-Ω test load?

7. Design a transistor add-on which would enable the reference voltage to remain constant under varying current flows to 1 A.

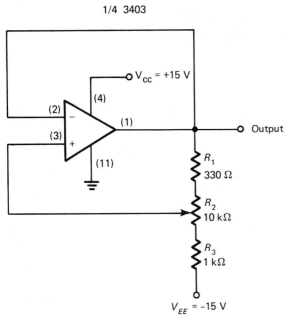

Fig. 10–1. **Positive voltage reference.**

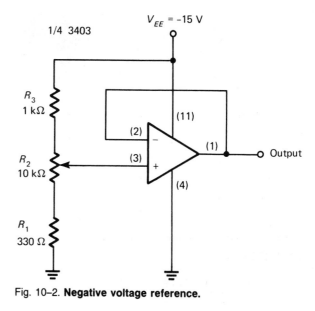

Fig. 10–2. **Negative voltage reference.**

SELF-TEST

Test your comprehension of the subject by answering the following questions.

1. In constant-voltage sources the voltage remains constant while the _____ can vary.
2. In a positive-voltage source the positive input to the amplifier is fed with a _____ voltage.
3. A constant-voltage source uses a circuit arrangement which is similar to a _____ -level detector.
4. The gain of a constant voltage source amplifier is _____ .
5. A negative constant voltage source requires a _____ signal source.

SELF-TEST ANSWERS
1. Current
2. Positive
3. Peak
4. Unity
5. Negative

11 CONSTANT-CURRENT SOURCES AND SINKS

OBJECTIVES

Upon completion of this experiment, construction of circuitry, testing, and evaluation of data, you will be able to:

1. *Design and construct current sources using linear integrated circuits*

2. *Test and evaluate constant-current source circuitry*

3. *Extend the capability of constant-current sources*

DISCUSSION

In this experiment regulation of constant-current sources and sinks is obtained by placing IC amplifiers in feedback loops of external transistors. Where constant current *sources* are desired, the external transistors are of the PNP variety. External NPN transistors are used to provide current *sinks*. Typical circuit designs include both fixed value and voltage variable configurations that can be either single or multiple source (or sink). The circuits consist of an operational amplifier which is used as a comparator. The positive input of the operational amplifier has a fixed or variable reference established by a resistive divider network. The negative input operates in the negative feedback

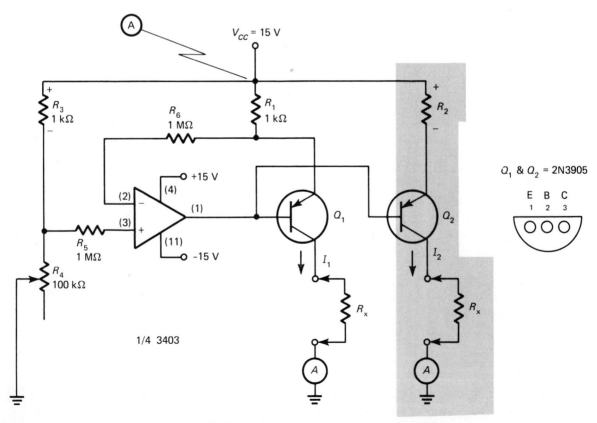

Fig. 11–1. **Constant-current source.**

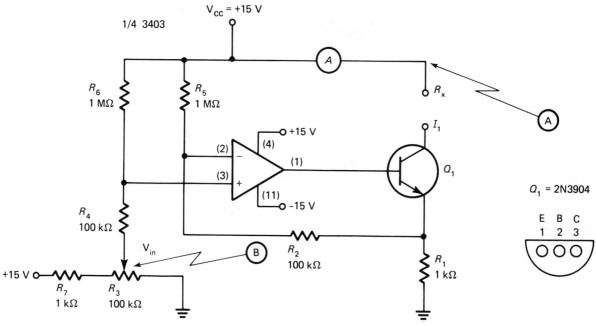

Fig. 11–2. **Constant-current sink.**

loop, thus causing the voltage drop across the emitter resistor of the external transistor to be maintained at the value of the reference voltage. Thus, the transistor emitter current is controlled and it is this same current that is available out of the collector.

A multiple-source constant-current configuration is presented in Fig. 11-1. The value of the output currents is controlled by the variable reference voltage established by the resistive divider network R_3 and R_4. This variable reference voltage is coupled to the positive input of the operational amplifier through R_5. Negative feedback is coupled to the negative input of the operational amplifier through R_6 which causes the voltage across R_1 to be maintained at the value of reference voltage. Since the value of R_1 together with the voltage developed across it determines the output current, it is referred to as the *current-control resistor*. For the second constant-current source (Q_2 circuitry), resistor R_2 is the current-controlling device. By scaling R_2, current I_2 can be made greater or less than current I_1. Figure 11-2 shows a configuration for a single output, voltage variable constant-current sink. The output current I_1 value is determined by the ratio of the input voltage (V_{in}) to the emitter resistance (R_1). This circuit will supply approximately 0 mA of output current for 0 V of DC input.

Typical applications for constant-current sources include maintaining lamp intensity in photoelectric circuits and in circuits where temperature changes or aging of components could cause a change in critical design parameters.

EQUATIONS

Current Source

$$I_1 = \frac{V_{ri}}{R_i} \tag{11-1}$$

$$I_2 = \frac{R_1}{R_2} \times I_1 \tag{11-2}$$

Current Sink

$$I_1 = \frac{1\ mA}{V\ DC\ input} \tag{11-3}$$

$$I_1 = \frac{V_{in}}{R_1} \tag{11-4}$$

MATERIALS REQUIRED

ACTIVE DEVICES:
   1 MC3403
   2 2N3905 Transistor
   1 2N3904 Transistor
RESISTORS: 5%, 1/4 W
   2 1 kΩ
   2 100 kΩ
   2 1 MΩ
   1 100-kΩ potentiometer
MISCELLANEOUS COMPONENTS:
   1 Socket, 14-pin
   2 Sockets, transistor

TEST INSTRUMENTS:
Oscilloscope, dual-trace, 5-in
Function generator, 10 Hz to MHz

Digital multimeter
Power supply, ± 15 V, 50 mA
Resistance decade boxes

TESTS AND MEASUREMENTS

Current Source

1. Construct the circuit of Fig. 11-1 using component values as shown, excluding R_2 and Q_2 (circuitry in screened area).

2. Connect a high-impedance voltmeter across R_3 and adjust R_4 for a reference potential of 1 V. At this setting of R_4, what is the value of V_{R1}? Compute the value of I_1 using equation (11-1).

3. Letting $R_x = 0$, measure and record the value of I_1. Letting $R_x = 100$ Ω, measure and record the value of I_1.

4. Determine the value of R_x at which I_1 can be no longer sustained at 1 mA. Explain why. (*Note:* The use of a resistance decade box or a 25-kΩ potentiometer will enable you to accomplish this test with ease.)

5. Referring to step 2 above, establish the reference potential at 2 V, determine the value of V_{R1}, the value of I_1, and the range over which R_x may vary.

6. Being careful *not* to disturb R_4, change R_1 to 500 Ω (two 1-kΩ resistors in parallel). What is the potential drop across the new value of R_1, the new constant current value, and the new range over which R_x can be allowed to vary?

7. Determine the range of constant-current output available by adjusting R_4 when $R_x = 0$ Ω, $R_1 = 1$ kΩ, and $V_{R3} = 1$ V.

8. The addition of the circuitry in the screened area provides for multiple sources of constant current from one controller. Add Q_2 and R_2 to the circuit as depicted after scaling R_2 to a value that would render $I_2 = 2I_1$. Compare the theoretical and measured results. (**NOTE:** Use the same parameters given in step 7 for making computations.)

Current Sink

9. Construct the current sink circuit of Fig. 11-2 using component values as indicated. Measure and record the voltage range available at test point B.

10. Letting $R_x = 0$ Ω, monitor test point B and the potential drop across R_1 (V_{R1}). Determine and record I_1 when $V_{in} = 1$ V DC.

11. Adjust R_4 for $V_{in} = 12$. Letting $R_x = 0$ Ω, measure and record I_1.

12. Compute the theoretical maximum range of R_x variation and let I_1 remain constant (step 11 circuit conditions apply). Using a resistance decade box, test the maximum range of R_x.

FOR FURTHER RESEARCH

13. Suppose that R_x is a lamp used in a photodetector system. On the basis of all tests conducted above, would the lamp brightness be held constant?

14. Could an additional output be made available from the circuit of Fig. 11-2? If so, provide the schematic and the equation for computing I_2.

SELF-TEST

Test your comprehension of the subject by answering the following questions.

1. In a constant-current source the current remains constant while the _____ resistance varies.

2. Constant current sources are typically used in _____ circuits.

3. The IC amplifier in a constant-current source acts as a _____ for controlling a transistor.

4. In Fig. 11-1, resistor _____ determines the current flow.

5. The current-carrying capacity of a current source can be increased by _____ another transistor with Q_1 in Fig. 11-1.

SELF-TEST ANSWERS

1. Load
2. Lamp loads, bridges, temperature
3. Constant voltage
4. R_1
5. Adding

12

ADDER SUBTRACTOR SUMMING AMPLIFIERS

OBJECTIVES

Upon completion of this experiment, construction of circuitry, testing, and evaluation of data, you will be able to:

1. *Design adder-type amplifiers such that two input voltages appear at the output of the amplifier as the sum*

2. *Design and evaluate amplifiers that provide the subtraction function*

3. *Apply such circuits to DC and AC voltages*

DISCUSSION

Adder- and/or subtractor-type circuits are used for computation as well as for the control of signals. Two or more DC input levels, plus or minus, can be handled by the circuit. Alternating-current signals can also be added in a similar manner. Variations of the circuit can be used, with comparators, for pulse detection and modulation. The circuit has a broad application.

Referring to Fig. 12-1, with A grounded (equal to 0), $V_1 + V_2 = V_{out}$ for $R_1 = R_2 = R_f$. *With A* connected to R_5 to ground (as shown), and if $R_5 = R_3 = R_4$, the following conditions exist:

1. $-V_1 + V_3 = V_{out} = V_1 + V_3$
2. $+V_1 - V_3 = -V_{out} = -V_1 - V_3$
3. $-V_1 - V_3 = +V_{out}$ (if $V_1 > V_3$) $= V_1 - V_3$
4. $+V_1 + V_3 = -V_{out}$ (if $V_1 > V_3$) $= V_1 + V_3$

The summing point B is a virtual ground and little or no current can flow from one input terminal to the other; hence each terminal is considered independent.

EQUATIONS

For A at ground—Summing Amplifier

$$V_{out} = -R_f \left(\frac{V_1}{R_1} + \frac{V_2}{R_2} \right) \qquad (12\text{-}1)$$

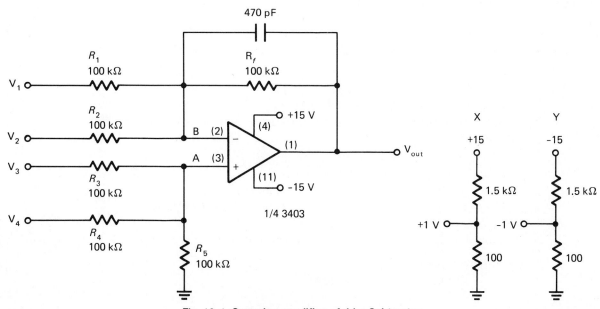

Fig. 12–1. **Summing amplifier—Adder-Subtractor.**

$$-V_{\text{out}} = \frac{V_1 R_f}{R_1} + \frac{V_2}{R_2} \qquad (12\text{-}2)$$

For A Not at ground—Difference Amplifier

$$V_{\text{out}} = \left(\frac{R_1 + R_2 + R_f}{R_3 + R_4 + R_5} \right)\left(\frac{R_5}{R_1} V_3 - V_4 \right)$$

$$- \left(\frac{R_f}{R_1} V_1 + V_2 \right) \qquad (12\text{-}3)$$

$$V_{\text{out}} \frac{R_5}{R_1} (V_3 - V_4)$$

$$- \frac{R_f}{R_1} (V_1 + V_2) \qquad (12\text{-}4)$$

where $R_1 = R_2 = R_3 = R_4$ and $R_f = R_5$.

MATERIALS REQUIRED

ACTIVE DEVICES:
  1 MC3403
RESISTORS: 5%, 1/4 W
  2 100 Ω
  2 1.5 kΩ
  6 100 kΩ
CAPACITORS: Disc, Mylar, electrolytic, 20%, 25 V
  1 470 pF
MISCELLANEOUS COMPONENTS:
  1 Socket, 14-pin
TEST INSTRUMENTS:
  Oscilloscope, dual-trace, 5-in
  Function generator, 10 Hz-to-1 MHz
  Digital multimeter
  Power supply ± 15 V, 50 mA

TESTS AND MEASUREMENTS

1. Construct the circuit shown in Fig. 12-1 using the indicated component values. Arrange the voltage dividers (circuits X and Y) as shown in order to obtain test voltages of approximately ± 1 V. Use these voltages for V_1 through V_4.

Adding ($A = 0$)
2. Determing V_{out} for $V_1 = -1$ V and $V_2 = -1$ V.

3. Determine V_{out} for $V_1 = +1$ V and $V_2 = +1$ V.

4. Determine V_{out} for $V_1 = -1$ V and $V_2 = +1$ V.

Subtracting ($A = 0$)
5. Determine V_{out} for $V_1 = +1$ V and $V_3 = -1$ V.

6. Determine V_{out} for $V_1 = -1$ V and $V_3 = +1$ V.

7. Determine V_{out} for $V_1 = -1$ V and $V_3 = -1$ V.

8. Letting $V_1 = +1$ V and $V_3 = -1$ V, change R_f to 470kΩ. Measure the value of V_{out} on an oscilloscope or meter and record the results.

9. Using Eq. (12-3), compute the value of V_{out} for step 8 and compare the results with the measured value (substitute the *actual* values of V_1 and V_2 in the equation).

10. Change all resistors in the circuit to 10kΩ. Repeat steps 2 and 5.

11. Change R_f to 47kΩ and repeat step 8.

Adding AC Signals
12. Change R_f to 10kΩ, $R_1 = 1$kΩ, and $R_2 = 2.2$kΩ. Ground point A. Feed V_1 with a 1=kH$_2$ sinewave of 100 m V peak-to-peak (p-p). Feed V_2 with a 100-Hz square wave adjusted to about 400 mV p=p. Draw the output waveshape at V_{out} and measure the amplitude of the output voltage.

FOR FURTHER RESEARCH
13. State at least two applications for these types of circuit.

14. Design a three-input adder to a comparator circuit. The amplifier should have a gain of 10.

SELF-TEST

Test your comprehension of the subject by answering the following questions. Refer to Fig. 12-1.

1. If $V_1 = +1$ V and $V_2 = +2$ V, the output voltage is _____V.

2. If $V_1 = -5$ V and $V_4 = +2$ V, the output is _____ V.

3. If $V_2 = +0.3$ V and $V_4 = +0.1$ V, the output is _____ V.

4. Inputs to V_1 and V_2 are phase _____, while inputs to V_3 and V_4 are _____.

5. If terminal 3 of the amplifier is grounded, the circuit is only a _____.

SELF-TEST ANSWERS
1. -3 **4.** Inverted, noninverted
2. $+7$ **5.** Summer
3. -0.2

13 COMPARATORS AS LAMP DRIVERS AND ADDERS

OBJECTIVES

Upon completion of this experiment, construction of circuitry, testing, and evaluation of data, you will be able to:

1. *Design, construct, and test comparator circuits to be used for lamp driving*

2. *Use a comparator/lamp driver so that two coincident incoming pulses must be present to drive the lamp to the on state*

3. *Apply this circuit concept to practical problems*

DISCUSSION

In this experiment you will use the comparator as an adder. Two signal input voltages will be added, compared with a reference, and when the sum is greater than the reference, the comparator will produce an output for driving a lamp. This type of circuit is utilized when it is desired to know if two events are occurring at the same time. The lamp shines as a visual indication while at the same time a control circuit can be activated.

Figure 13-1 shows a comparator used as an adder to drive a light-emitting diode (LED) on when the sum of its inputs is greater than the reference. The comparator's reference voltage is determined by R_2. In this experiment two signals, a square wave and a sine wave, are fed to the inputs V_2 and V_1, respectively. Since the square wave is higher in amplitude, R_5 is made larger than R_4.

To turn the lamp on when the positive halves of both signals arrive together, the reference voltage of the comparator is adjusted so that *only* the summed signal will be sufficient to produce an output at pin 1. The coincidental appearance of both signals will produce a positive pulse at the output of the comparator. Since the output is normally low, transistor Q_1 is biased off. When a positive pulse appears at the base, Q_1 is biased on and a part of the collector current I_C flows through the LED. Resistor R_7 limits the current through the

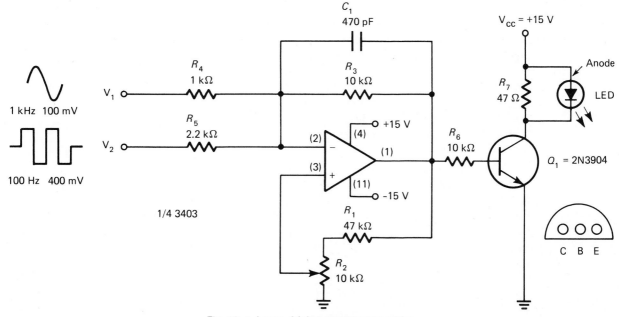

Fig. 13–1. **Lamp-driving comparator-adder.**

LED by providing a parallel path to V_{CC}. *Capacitor C_1 provides stability and also limits the amplifier's frequency response.*

EQUATIONS

Refer to experiment 12.

MATERIALS REQUIRED

ACTIVE DEVICES:
1 MC3403
1 2N3904 transistor
1 1.7-V light-emitting diode (LED)

RESISTORS: 5%, ¼ W
1 47 Ω
1 1 kΩ
1 2.2 kΩ
2 10 kΩ
1 47 kΩ
1 10-kΩ potentiometer

CAPACITORS: disc, Mylar, electrolytic, 20%, 25 V
1 470 pF

MISCELLANEOUS COMPONENTS:
1 Socket, 14-pin

TEST INSTRUMENTS:
Oscilloscope, dual-trace, 5-in
Function generator, 10 Hz-to-1 MHz
Digital multimeter
Power supply, ±15 V, 50 mA

TESTS AND MEASUREMENTS

---

1. Construct the circuit shown in Fig. 13-1, using component values as shown. Ensure that the LED is properly connected (the cathode is usually indicated by a longer lead).

2. To establish the reference level, ground both V_1 and V_2 inputs, remove Q_1, and adjust R_2 to obtain a range of -1.07 to -1.10 V DC at pin 3. Remove the grounds at the inputs and reinsert transistor Q_1 into the circuit.

3. Feed a 1-kHz sine wave at 100 mV to input V_1, feed a 100-Hz square wave at 400 mV to input V_2, and measure and record the output wave of the comparator. (NOTE: Adjustment of R_2 may be necessary to obtain *precise* triggering.)

4. Determine the resting potential of pin 1 of the 3403. This is the voltage that maintains transistor Q_1 in an "off" state. (NOTE: This measurement is accomplished with the comparator in a quiescent state.)

5. Determine the level of signal appearing *only* at V_1 (1-kHz sine wave) needed to trigger the comparator. How much signal appearing *only* at input V_2 (100-Hz square wave) is required to trigger the comparator?

FOR FURTHER RESEARCH

6. State at least two applications for such circuits as the one studied in this experiment.

SELF-TEST

Test your comprehension of the subject by answering the following questions.

1. In a comparator, one input is set to a _____ level while the other amplifier input is controlled by the incoming signal.

2. When the comparator's threshold level is passed, a _____ pulse is produced.

3. An NPN transistor is required in Fig. 13-1 since the comparator's output goes _____.

4. The input circuit of Fig. 13-1 is a _____.

5. To illuminate a LED, the anode must be _____ and the cathode, _____.

SELF-TEST ANSWERS
1. Reference
2. Positive
3. Positive
4. Summer
5. Positive, negative

14 INTEGRATORS

OBJECTIVES

Upon completion of this experiment, construction of circuitry, testing, and evaluation of data, you will be able to:

1. *Construct, test, and evaluate integrator circuits using operational amplifiers*

2. *Evaluate the use of integrating circuits for control systems and instrumentation*

3. *Apply the concepts learned to practical circuits*

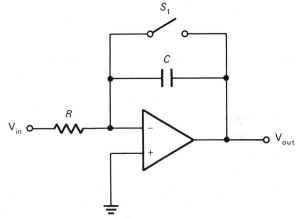

Fig. 14–1. **Basic integrator circuit.**

DISCUSSION

The term *integrator* should not be confused with *integrated circuit* (IC). An integrator performs the mathematical operation of integration, which is, essentially, to find the area under the curve generated by the input waveform. The latter term (IC) defines a method of interconnecting associated circuit elements inseparably on a substrate. Refer to Fig. 14-1. As the input signal (V_{in}) varies, the value over small intervals of time (dt) is determined, dependent on the RC time constant. The output voltage V_{out} is expressed mathematically:

$$V_{out} = \int_0^T V_{in}\,dt$$

When the input signal is a square wave, the output voltage will be a triangular wave, as shown in Fig. 14-2. When the input signal is a sine wave, the output voltage also will be a sine wave, but shifted 90° in phase (see Fig. 14-3). Switch 1 (Fig. 14-1) provides a means of establishing initial circuit conditions. In practical circuits this can be accomplished by using a relay in very slow circuits or an electronic switch for more rapid applications.

The time constant of the integrator is critical. As a general rule of thumb, it is safe to make the time constant not less than the period of the expected input waveform.

Another important design consideration in the use of

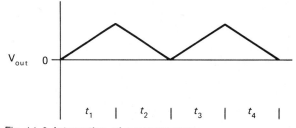

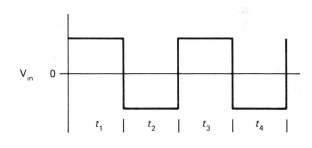

Fig. 14–2. **Integration of a square wave.**

an operational amplifier as an integrator is the provision of DC feedback. Because of this feedback, the offset error voltage cannot charge the capacitor continuously up to the amplifier limits. Normally the DC feedback is provided by shunting the integrating capacitor with a resistor. The resulting RC time con-

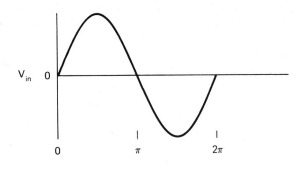

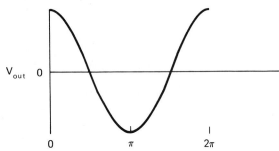

Fig. 14–3. **Integration of a sine wave.**

EQUATIONS

$$R_1 = R_2$$

for minimum offset error due to bias current   (14-1)

$$f_{out} = \frac{1}{6.28 R_1 C_1} \qquad (14\text{-}2)$$

$$V_{out} = \frac{1}{R_1 C_1} \int_0^T V_{in}\, dt \qquad (14\text{-}3)$$

$$V_{out} \cong \frac{X_{C1}}{R_1} \qquad \text{for frequencies below } f_c \qquad (14\text{-}4)$$

MATERIALS REQUIRED

ACTIVE DEVICES:
   1 MC3403
RESISTORS: 5%, 1/4 W
   2 10 kΩ
   1 100 kΩ
CAPACITORS: disc, Mylar, electrolytic, 20%, 25 V
   1 0.047 μF
MISCELLANEOUS COMPONENTS:
   1 Socket 14-Pin
TEST INSTRUMENTS:
   Oscilloscope, dual-trace, 5 in
   Function generator, 10 Hz to 1 MHz
   Digital multimeter
   Power supply, ±15 V, 50 mA
   Capacitance decade box

stant is substantially longer than the periods for the frequencies of interest. The DC gain of the circuit will be limited by the feedback resistor; however, the effect of the resistor on the gain becomes negligible at frequencies above the corner frequency (f_c) because of the capacitor paralleling it.

For the operational amplifier integrator, the output voltage will be equal to the integral of the input waveform, divided by the RC time constant.

TESTS AND MEASUREMENTS

1. Construct the circuit shown in Fig. 14-4 using component values indicated. Measure and record static voltages.

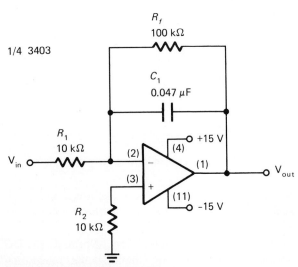

Fig. 14–4. **An integrator amplifier.**

2. Apply a 0.5-V DC signal to the input, measure V_{out}, and determine the DC gain of the circuit in decibels.

3. Apply a 1-V DC signal at the input, measure V_{out}, and compute the gain of the circuit in decibels. While observing the output, remove the DC feedback resistor R_f. Describe and explain what you observed.

4. Apply a 1-kHz square wave of 5 V p-p to the input. Measure and record the output voltage and waveform. Using Eq. (14-4), determine the value of V_{out} and compare it with the measured value.

5. What is the amplitude of V_{out} when a 5-kHz, 5-V p-p square wave is fed to the input?

6. Feed the input with a triangular voltage of 5 V p-p at 1 kHz. Measure and record the output voltage amplitude and waveform.

7. Apply a sine wave of 5 V p-p at 1 kHz to the input. Measure and record the output voltage amplitude and waveform.

(NOTE: Further use of this circuit will be made in the following experiment. *Do not disassemble at this time.*)

Test your comprehension of the subject by answering the following questions.

1. If a square wave is integrated, the output will be a _____ wave.
2. An integrator _____ the area under the curve of the input waveshape.
3. The gain of the integrator in Fig. 14-4 is determined by the ratio of _____ and _____.
4. The gain of the amplifier in Fig. 14-4, set by R_f and R_1, is effective _____ the corner frequency of the amplifier.
5. If a chain of pulses is fed to an integrator, the output will be the _____ of the pulses.

SELF-TEST ANSWERS
1. Triangle
2. Sums
3. R_f and R_1
4. Below
5. Average

EXPERIMENT **15** DIFFERENTIATORS

OBJECTIVES

Upon completion of this experiment, construction of circuitry, testing, and performance evaluation of data, you will be able to:

1. *Construct, test, and evaluate differentiator circuits using operational amplifiers*

2. *Evaluate the use of differentiators for instrumentation, computers, and other sophisticated applications*

3. *Apply the concepts learned to practical circuits*

DISCUSSION

Differentiation is the determination of the instantaneous rate of change of a function. The slope of a line tangent to the point of interest on the graph of the function represents the rate of change. An electronic differentiator using an operational amplifier is shown in Fig. 15-1. This circuit computes the negative of $dV_{in} dt$ (since the inverting input is used) as long as the RC time constant is proper.

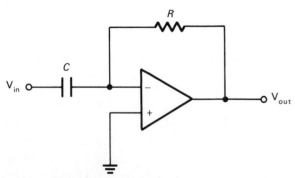

Fig. 15–1. **The basic differentiator.**

An initial requirement of a differentiator is that it be designed to respond only to *changes* in the input (the rate of change of a constant is 0). To accomplish this requirement, a capacitor is placed in series with the inverting input of the operational amplifier. For the ideal situation, if the input voltage function were to change *instantaneously* (i.e., have a 0 transition time), the *true* differentiator output would be infinitely large. The ideal or true differentiator cannot be achieved; moreover, "real-world" signals do not have instantaneous transition times. Square waves have the fastest transition times available, but even they are finite. Nevertheless, many tests can be performed on the practical differentiator with the use of available real-world input signals.

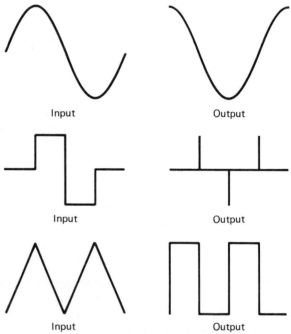

Fig. 15–2. **Input-output wave shapes of a differentiator.**

Aside from the mathematical operations associated with calculus, one way of describing a differentiator is to examine its effects on various types of waveform (see Fig. 15-2). This effect is a distortion of the wave; the amount of distortion is dependent on the value of the circuit's time constant compared to the period of the waveform. However, a differentiator cannot alter the shape of a pure sine wave. Refer to Fig. 15-2. A sine wave, when fed through the differentiator, will produce the cosine wave at the output (a 90° phase shift). A cosine input signal, on the other hand, will produce the "minus sine" wave (an inversion) at the output. The triangular wave results in a square wave when it is differentiated. Square waves are affected in a special way: a bipolar train of sharp pulses results (examine the waveform and you will see why).

Since a differentiator is designed to respond only to *changes* in the input signal, the time constant of the circuit is of considerable importance. Figure 15-3 shows the outputs of a short-time-constant circuit for two sawtooth input waves. The slope of the trailing edge on each waveform is greater than that of the leading edge. As the transition time of the input waveform decreases (i.e., the interval from 1 to 2 is shortened), negative peaks of the output voltage increase correspondingly. Generally, the RC time constant of a differentiator is about 10 percent of the period of the expected waveform.

$$f_c = \frac{1}{6.28R_1C_1} \qquad (15\text{-}2)$$

$$f_h = \frac{1}{6.28R_3C_1} = \frac{1}{6.28R_1C_2} \qquad (15\text{-}3)$$

$$f_c \ll f_h \ll f_{\text{unity gain}} \qquad (15\text{-}4)$$

MATERIALS REQUIRED

ACTIVE DEVICES:
 1 MC3403
RESISTORS: 5%, 1/4 W
 1 270 Ω
 2 10 kΩ
CAPACITORS: disc, Mylar, electrolytic, 20%, 25 V
 1 0.001 μF
 1 0.1 μF
MISCELLANEOUS COMPONENTS:
 1 Socket, 14-pin
TEST INSTRUMENTS:
 Oscilloscope, dual-trace, 5-in
 Function generator, 10 Hz to 1 MHz
 Digital multimeter
 Power supply, ±15 V, 50 mA

EQUATIONS

$$V_{\text{out}} = R_1C_1 \frac{dV_{\text{in}}}{dt} \qquad (15\text{-}1)$$

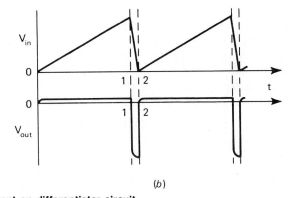

Fig. 15–3. **Effects of time constant on differentiator circuit.**

TESTS AND MEASUREMENTS

1. Construct the circuit shown in Fig. 15-4 using component values indicated. Measure and record static voltages. (**NOTE:** This circuit is to be configured in conjunction with the circuitry of Experiment 14.)

2. Feed the input with a 0.5-V p-p 1-kHz signal (be careful not to saturate the amplifier). Measure and record the output voltage amplitude and waveshape.

3. Apply a 0.5-V p-p 1-kHz triangular wave at V_{in}. Measure and record the output voltage and waveform.

4. Apply a 0.5-V p-p 1-kHz sine wave at the input. Measure and record the output voltage and waveform.

5. Explain why the amplitude of the output-voltage waveforms in steps 3 and 4 are less than that of step 2.

6. Use the parallel combination of $R = 4.7\text{k}\Omega$ and $C = 0.22$ μF to interconnect the output of the integrator (Experiment 14) to the input of the differentiator (see Fig. 15-5).

a. Apply a square wave of 1 kHz at 0.5 V p-p to the integrator input. What is the waveform reproduced at V_{out} of the differentiator?

b. Feed a triangular wave of 1 kHz at 0.5 V p-p to the integrator. Was V_{out} of the differentiator a 1-kHz triangular wave?

c. Use a 1-kHz sine wave as the input to the integrator. Was V_{out} of the differentiator a reproduction of the integrator input signal?

7. Would you expect the results to be similar to those obtained in step 6 if the differentiator and integrator were reversed?

FOR FURTHER RESEARCH
8. Give several applications for a differentiator.

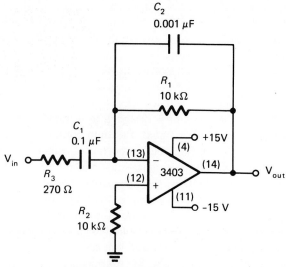

Fig. 15–4. **A differentiating amplifier.**

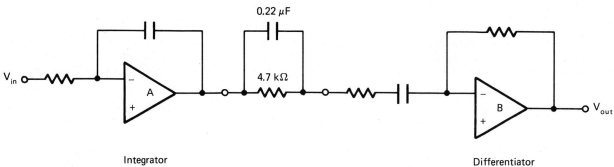

Fig. 15–5. **Cascading an integrator and differentiator.**

SELF-TEST

Test your comprehension of the subject by answering the following questions.

1 What is the equation for computing the circuit's time constant?

2 If a square-wave positive pulse is fed into a differentiator, the output will be a _____ .

3. The leading edge of a pulse represents the _____ frequency portion of the wave.

4. A triangular wave, when differentiated, produces a _____ wave.

5. The time constant of a differentiator should always be _____ than the pulse period.

SELF-TEST ANSWERS
1. $T = RC$
2. Spiked pulses
3. High
4. Square
5. Less

EXPERIMENT **16**

MULTIPLYING WITH FOUR-QUADRANT INTEGRATED CIRCUITS

OBJECTIVES

Upon completion of this experiment, construction of circuitry, testing, and performance evaluation of data, you will be able to:

1. *Construct, test, and evaluate a unique integrated circuit designed as a multiplier to provide a multiplication function*

2. *Test and evaluate level shift operational amplifiers used with multipliers and evaluate both AC and DC operation*

3. *Apply the concepts learned to other functions such as divide, square, and square root*

DISCUSSION

The MC1495 chip is designed to perform mathematical functioning. In the experiment the multiplication function is evaluated. Some functions provided by this chip are similar to those of the MC1496, which is used in telecommunications. Complete details on operations appear in Motorola applications notes AN-489 and in the data sheets provided in Appendix A. The MC1495 is a monolithic, four-quadrant multiplier which has application in circuits that must perform multiply, divide, square, square-root, or modulate functions. Certainly, because the MC1495 is so versatile, it has many other applications, such as phase detection, demodulation, and electronic gain control.

The error in linearity is 4 percent or less with the MC1495 and under 2 percent with the MC1595. The inputs (two) can handle ± 10 V, while scaling (scale factor K) is adjustable. Figure 16-1 shows the circuit design incorporated. The differential amplifiers Q_1 and Q_2 handle the Y input, while Q_3 and Q_4 handle the X input. Mixing is provided by amplifiers Q_5, Q_6, Q_7, and Q_8. Differential gain control is provided for each set of amplifiers, X and Y, by external resistors connected to pins 5 and 6 for Y and 10 and 11 for X. Current flow adjusting and balancing (scale-factor adjustment) is

provided by external resistors connected to pins 3 and 13. The output from both X and Y amplifiers is taken from pins 2 and 14 *(KXY)*. The positive voltage V_{CC} is applied to pin 1, while the negative voltage V_{EE} is applied to pin 7. The chip is designed for ± 15 V of operation.

In operation, three controls are provided for nulling out offset currents (see Fig. 16-2): Y (by adjusting potentiometer P_1), X (by adjusting potentiometer P_2), and output (by adjusting potentiometer P_4). Scaling is provided by adjusting the current flow of I_3 in relation to I_{13} with potentiometer P_3. The added operational amplifier provides DC level shifting (1741, MC3403, or similar can be used). While the input voltage to X and Y can be 10 V, voltage dividers are provided so that 5 V is the voltage level. By adjusting these resistor values, voltages above 10 V can be used.

The method for selecting component values is presented in the technical notes for the MC1495 in Appendix A (see general design procedures). Assuming these values to be correct, emphasis is placed on testing and evaluation of how the circuit performs and how it can be used and applied.

Level Shifting

For DC applications, such as multiply, divide, and square-root functions, it is usually desirable to connect the differential output to a single-ended output voltage referenced to ground. The output of the operational amplifier level shifter follows the current $I_2 - I_{14}$, where $V_{out} = (I_2 - I_{14})RL$. The amplifier used must have a low-input current, high-input resistance, and good common-mode rejection (CMR).

Offset and Scale Factor

The transistors and resistors within the IC have been closely matched. Differences are present, however, and external adjustments are needed to correct X and Y offset as well as output offset. Potentiometers P_1, P_2, and P_4 are used to set these offsets to zero. For DC operations one or all three of the controls may be required, but some may be eliminated for AC. In the

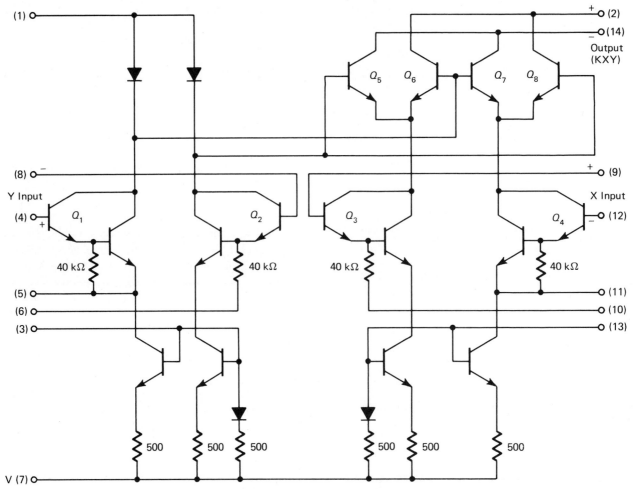

Fig. 16–1. **Circuit diagram of an MC1495L multiplier.**

experiment circuit the power supplies are fairly well regulated, and a simpler balancing arrangement can be used.

The scale factor K, set by P_3, controls the I_3 current which inversely sets the scale factor K. The value of K will be determined and used in most DC calculations. Scaling permits the DC functions to be carried out within the limits of the supply voltages. Suppose, for example, 10 V was applied to both the X and Y inputs for multiplication. The output would have to be 100 V, which is beyond the supply voltage available. By scaling, with $K = 1/10$, the output is set to 10 V. The scaling factor K, set by P_3, is used when the operations are not easily handled.

Linearity

The output $V_{out} = KV_x V_y$, where V'_x and V'_y at the input can also be scaled by voltage dividers R_1, R_2 and R_3, R_4 as seen in the circuit shown in Fig. 16-2. The circuit uses gain resistors R_x and R_y, which are different in value. Increasing R_y improves the Y linearity; the slight reduction in R_x does not materially affect X linearity while avoiding a significant increase in R_L to maintain K at the same value. If the power supply is

not well regulated, the offset controls P_1 and P_2 should be operated from a Zener-regulated supply. The methods and procedures of adjusting the amplifier's offset and K factor is presented under the "Tests and Measurements" section in this experiment. When required in the next experiment, reference should also be made to these procedures. The MC1495 chip is unique and valuable in its contribution to electronic circuitry. In this experiment it is considered as a multiplier.

EQUATIONS

$$V_{out} = K (V_x - V_y) \qquad (16\text{-}1)$$

where: V_x, V_y = pins 9 and 4, respectively

$$K = \frac{V_{out}}{V_x - V_y} = \frac{2R_L}{R_x R_y I_3} \qquad (16\text{-}2)$$

where: $I_3 \cong 1$ mA

$$R_L \cong 40 \text{ k}\Omega$$

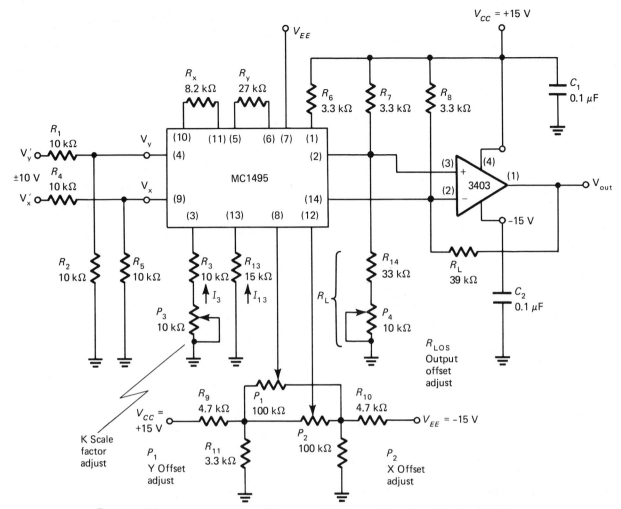

Fig. 16–2. **Wiring diagram of a multiplier circuit with operational amplifier level shifting.**

$$V_{out} = K \, (V'_x \times V'_y)R_K \qquad (16\text{-}3)$$

where: V_{out} = output due to multiplier input

R_K ratio of voltage divider at each input to multiplier

V'_x, V'_y = full voltage at inputs X and Y

$$R_K = \frac{V_x}{V'_x} \qquad (16\text{-}4)$$

$$\frac{V_y}{V'_y}$$

EXAMPLE: Let $V = V = +10$ V DC, let $K = 0.4$, and let each voltage divider divide the voltage by 50 percent at the inputs. Determine V_{out} at the output of the operational amplifier.

1. Solving for R_K: $R_K = \left(\dfrac{V_x}{V}\right)\left(\dfrac{V_y}{V}\right)$

$$= 0.5 \times 0.5 = 0.25$$

2. Solving for V_{out}: $V_{out} = K(V \, V) \, R_K$

$$= 0.4 \times 10 \times 10 \times 0.25$$

$$= 10 \text{ V}$$

MATERIALS REQUIRED

ACTIVE DEVICES:
 1 MC1495
 1 MC3403
RESISTORS: 5%, 1/4 W
 5 3.3 kΩ
 1 33 kΩ
 2 4.7 kΩ
 1 39 kΩ
 1 8.2 kΩ
 5 10 kΩ
 1 15 kΩ
 1 10 kΩ
 1 27 kΩ
 2 100-kΩ potentiometers
CAPACITORS: disc, Mylar, electrolytic, 20%, 25 V
 2 0.1MF
MISCELLANEOUS COMPONENTS
 2 Sockets, 14-pin
TEST INSTRUMENTS:
 Oscilloscope, dual-trace, 5-in
 Function generator, 10 Hz to 1 MHz
 Digital multimeter
 Power supply, ±15 V, 50 mA

Procedures

The first tests, after the circuit of Fig. 16-2 has been constructed using the component values shown, involve setting of the offset (os) controls P_1, P_2, and P_4. The manufacturer's suggested procedure is used to null the offsets and set the scale factor for the multiply mode.

1. X Input offset:

   a. Apply a 1-kHz, 5-V p-p sine wave to the Y input (pin 4).

   b. Ground the X input (pin 9).

   c. Adjust the X offset potentiometer, P_2, for an AC null at the output.

2. Y Input offset:

   a. Apply a 1-kHz, 5 V p-p sine wave signal to the X input (pin 9).

   b. Ground the Y input (pin 4).

   c. Adjust the Y offset potentiometer, P_1, for an AC null at the output.

3. Output offset:

   a. Ground both the V'_x and V'_y inputs.

   b. Adjust output offset potentiometer, P_4, until the output $V_{out} = 0$ V DC.

4. Scale factor:

   a. Apply $+10$ V DC to both V'_x and V'_y inputs.

   b. Adjust potentiometer P_3 to obtain $+10$ V DC at the output V_{out}.

5. Repeat steps 1 through 4 as necessary.

6. Measure and record all static voltages (short V and V to ground). Then measure and record currents I_3 and I_{13}.

7. Calculate the scaling factor K using the current for I_3 obtained in step 6 above.

8. Apply $+10$ V DC to the V'_x and V'_y inputs. Compute R_K and V_{out} and compare the values obtained with the measured values. (**NOTE:** Obtain the $+10$-V-DC voltage by making use of a voltage divider network if a separate DC source is not available.)

9. Apply $+10$ V DC to the V'_x input and -10 V DC to the V'_y input. Compute V_{out} and compare the value obtained with the measured value. (**NOTE:** Where the calculated and measured values of V_{out} differ significantly, recheck your null and scaling settings prior to proceeding to step 10.)

10. Apply -5 V DC to V'_x and $+10$ V DC to V'_y. What is the value of V_{out}?

11. Apply -5 V DC to V'_x and -10 V DC to V'_y. Measure and record V_{out}.

12. If the input voltages applied to the multiplier in steps 10 and 11 were reversed, would you expect different results?

13. To familiarize yourself with operation of the chip as a multiplier, try various combinations of DC input voltages and compare the measured and computed values of V_{out}. Determine whether the *product* of the inputs when multiplied by the scaling factor K and voltage ratio R_K has been obtained. Even with careful matching of transistor emitter junctions in the MC1495L chip (typically within 1 mV), an output error can occur. This output error is comprised of X input offset voltage, Y input offset voltage, and output offset voltage. Adjustment to 0 of these errors is accomplished with potentiometers P_1, P_2, and P_4. For most DC applications, all three offset potentiometers will be required to achieve accuracy.

14. To achieve the squaring function, it is necessary to tie the two inputs together. For this operational mode, the output voltage follows the equation $V_{out} = KV^2$ (excluding the ratio of the voltage divider at each input). Additionally, a slightly different procedure is used to null the offset for AC applications. Use the following AC adjustment procedure:

   a. Tie V'_x and V'_y together. Apply a 1-kHz, 10-V-p-p sine wave at the input.

   b. Monitor V_{out} by using an oscilloscope and an AC voltmeter.

   c. Adjust P_3 (scaling factor) for maximum voltage on the AC voltmeter while observing the waveform on the Oscilloscope.

   d. Adjust P_1 for *equal peaks* on the oscilloscope OR the lowest reading on the AC voltmeter.

   e. Ground the input and adjust P_4 (output offset) such that $V_{out} = 0$ V DC.

   f. Repeat steps **a** through **e** as necessary.

15. Apply a 2-kHz, 10-V-p-p sine wave to the input; measure and record the amplitude and frequency of V_{out}.

16. Compute the value of K for this setting of P_3.

17. Apply a 3-V-p-p, 4-kHz sine wave to the input and compare the computed and measured values of V_{out}.

FOR FURTHER RESEARCH

18. Read Motorola application notes AN-489, Analysis and Basic Operation of MC1595 and technical data notes in the Appendix.

19. Check for the similarity of the MC1595 with the operation of the MC1596.

Test your comprehension of the subject by answering the following questions.

1. If the input signal voltage is too large _____ is necessary
2. Resistors R_x and R_y control the _____.
3. The MC3403 amplifier provides _____ level shifting.
4. The multiplier can handle both DC and AC signals (true or false).
5. The circuit of Fig. 16-2 will provide a squaring function if both inputs are connected together (true or false).

SELF-TEST ANSWERS

1. Scaling
2. Gain
3. DC
4. True
5. True

17 AC-TO-DC CONVERTERS

OBJECTIVES

Upon completion of this experiment, construction of circuitry, testing, and evaluation of data, you will be able to:

1. *Construct and evaluate AC-to-DC converters using operational amplifiers*

2. *Evaluate circuitry designed to overcome diode conduction threshold*

3. *Evaluate both half-wave and full-wave operational amplifier rectifier circuits*

DISCUSSION

The semiconductor diodes available today are close to ideal devices but have severe limitations in low-level applications. Silicon diodes have a 0.6-V threshold which must be overcome before any appreciable conduction can occur. When the diode is placed in the feedback loop of an operational amplifier, threshold voltage is divided by the open loop gain of the amplifier. Millivolt signal rectification becomes possible with virtual elimination of threshold.

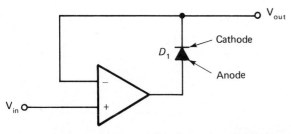

Fig. 17–1. **Basic circuit for elimination of threshold voltage of a diode.**

The basic circuit configuration for eliminating diode threshold potential is shown in Fig. 17-1. A positive voltage at the *noninverting* (+) input causes the output to swing positive. Once the voltage at the output of the operational amplifier reaches 0.6 V, D_1 becomes forward biased and conducts. The negative feedback through D_1 forces the *inverting* input (−) to follow the

noninverting input, and the circuit will act as a voltage follower for positive signals. When a negative signal is applied at the *non*inverting input, the output of the operational amplifier also becomes negative and D_1 is cut off; thus no current will flow in the load (neglecting bias current of the operational amplifier).

Generally, the open-loop gain of an operational amplifier is in the thousands, producing a 0.6-V output with microvolt-level input signals; thus the diode threshold for conduction has been greatly reduced.

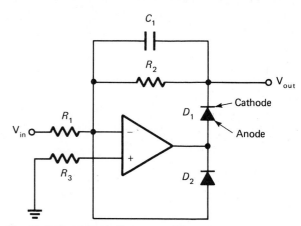

Fig. 17–2. **Precision half-wave rectifier.**

A precision, high-performance half-wave rectifier is shown in Figure 17-2. This circuit is easily extended for full-wave rectification, and its function is somewhat different from that of the circuit shown in Fig. 17-1. The input signal is applied through R_1 to the inverting input terminal of the amplifier. When the input is negative, diode D_1 is forward biased and develops an output across R_2; the gain being in accordance with the ratio of R_2 to R_1. For a positive input signal, D_1 is cut off and there is no output. But the negative feedback is then supplied through diode D_2. This action prevents the amplifier from becoming saturated as a result of an "open" feedback loop, and the negative output voltage swing is held to about 0.7 V.

If a second operational amplifier is added to the circuit, the half-wave rectifier will be converted to a full-wave rectifier. Refer to Fig. 17-3. The output of A_1

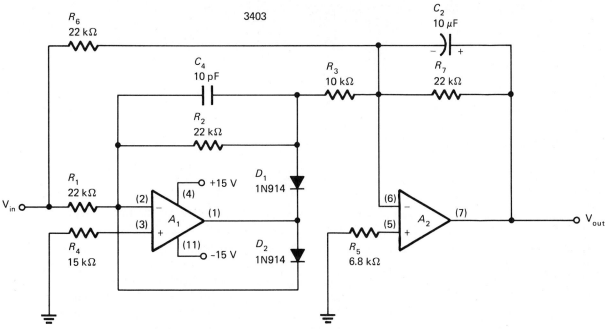

Fig. 17–3. **Full-wave precision rectifier.**

(half-wave rectifier) is connected to the inverting input of A_2. Amplifier A_2 sums the half-wave rectified signal and input signal (applied through R_6) to provide a full-wave output. When V_i is negative, A_1 output is zero, and no signal is applied through R_3 to A_2. For positive input signals, the currents through R_3 and R_6 are summed at the inverting input of A_2. Filtering to obtain a pure DC output is accomplished by capacitor C_2. The filter time constant is R_7C_2, must be much greater than the maximum period of the input signal.

EQUATIONS

Unfiltered

$$V_{out} = R_7 \left(\frac{V_{in}}{R_3} - \frac{V_{in}}{R_6} \right) \qquad (17\text{-}1)$$

Filtered

$$V_{out} = 0.707 V_{in,\,peak} \qquad (17\text{-}2)$$

MATERIALS REQUIRED

ACTIVE DEVICES:
  1 MC3403;
  2 IN914 Diodes
RESISTORS: 5%, 14 W
  1 6.8 kΩ
  1 10 kΩ
  1 15 kΩ
  4 22 kΩ
CAPACITORS: disc, Mylar, electrolytic, 20%, 25 V
  1 10 pF
  1 10 MF
MISCELLANEOUS COMPONENTS:
  1 Socket, 14-pin
TEST INSTRUMENTS:
  Oscilloscope, dual trace, 5-in
  Function generator, 10 Hz to 1 MHz
  Digital multimeter
  Power supply, $\pm$15 V, 50 mA

TESTS AND MEASUREMENTS

1. Construct the circuit shown in Fig. 17-3 using component values as indicated. Measure and record static voltages. (NOTE: Use *sine wave* signals only for steps 2 through 8.)

2. Disconnect capacitor C_2 and resistor R_6. Let $V_{in} = 0.1$ V p-p at 1 kHz. Measure and record the amplitude and waveform of V_{out}. Is the output a half-wave or a full-wave voltage?

3. Reconnect resistor R_6 and maintain $V_{in} = 0.1$ V p-p at 1 kHz. Record the amplitude and wave form of V_{out}. Is the output a half-wave or a full-wave voltage?

4. Replace capacitor C_2. Measure and record the output voltage V_{out} while keeping $V_{in} = 0.1$ V p-p at 1 kHz. Is the output DC?

5. Maintain $V_{in} = 0.1$ V p-p and vary the frequency

from 100 Hz to 1 kHz. Does the DC output level change?

6. Increase the amplitude of V_{in} to 0.5 V p-p @ 1 kHz. What is the value of V_{out}?

8. What is the value of V_{out} with a 1-kHz input of 0.15 V p-p, 0.25 V p-p, and 0.5 V p-p? Do the DC output values follow Eq. (17-2)?

FOR FURTHER RESEARCH

7. Substitute a 0.05-μF capacitor for C_2. What effect does this have on the output at 1 kHz?

SELF-TEST

Test your comprehension of the subject by answering the following questions.

1. The turn-on voltage of most silicon diodes is _____ volts.

2. If a diode is placed in the feedback loop of a high-gain amplifier, it will break down in the _____ range.

3. In Fig. 17-3, amplifier A_1 provides _____ -wave rectification.

4. The overall circuit of Fig. 17-3 provides _____ -wave rectification and filtering.

5. The time constant of $R_7 - C_2$ should be _____ than the time period of the incoming signal voltage.

SELF-TEST ANSWERS

1. 0.6
2. Millivolt or microvolt
3. Half
4. Full
5. Greater

EXPERIMENT 18 BRIDGE AMPLIFIERS

OBJECTIVES

Upon completion of this experiment, construction of circuitry, testing, and evaluation of data, you will be able to:

1. *Use an operational amplifier and thermistor for designing, building, and testing temperature measuring amplifiers*

2. *Design a strain gage circuit with operational amplifiers for measuring strain*

3. *Arrange bridge amplifier circuitry for use with other transducers*

DISCUSSION

A Wheatstone bridge circuit is used in this experiment. One leg of the bridge is the transducer for measuring temperature, pressure, strain, and so on, and the other legs are resistors. A high-gain, high-input-impedance operational amplifier is used for measuring the voltage generated by the unbalancing of the bridge. A four-legged bridge is shown in Fig. 18-1, and a meter is shown indicating the null balance. Figure 18-2 shows

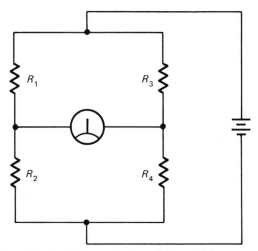

Fig. 18–1. **Circuit diagram of a Wheatstone bridge.**

the same circuit with one resistor (R_2) replaced with a temperature- or strain-sensitive resistive device. As a thermistor has a negative temperature coefficient of resistance, its resistance would decrease with increasing temperature, thus causing an increase in current in the circuit.

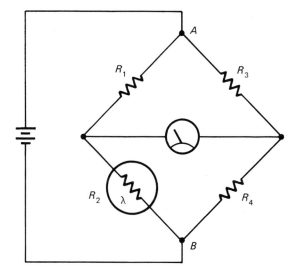

Fig. 18–2. **Transducer bridge circuit.**

Since the meter in these types of circuit must be very sensitive, are subject to damage, and are costly, an amplifier and a standard milliammeter can be used more effectively. Figure 18-3 shows one such circuit. The gain of the amplifier is determined by the ratio R_5/R_3. The larger is the value of R_5, the higher is the gain and sensitivity of the metering. Capacitor C_1 limits the frequency response and prevents amplifier oscillation. The legs of the bridge are R_1/R_2 and R_3/R_4. At balance, the voltage across R_2 equals the voltage across R_4, and the meter on the output reads 0. Potentiometer R_6 is used to reduce the sensitivity of the meter and also to calibrate the meter range. A 1-mA meter could be calibrated to 100° full scale. The meter can be 0 to 10 mA [usually available in a volt-ohm-milliammeter (VOM) instrument]. The thermistor used is 100kΩ. For lower thermistor resistance values or strain gauges, lower values of bridge resistors would be used.

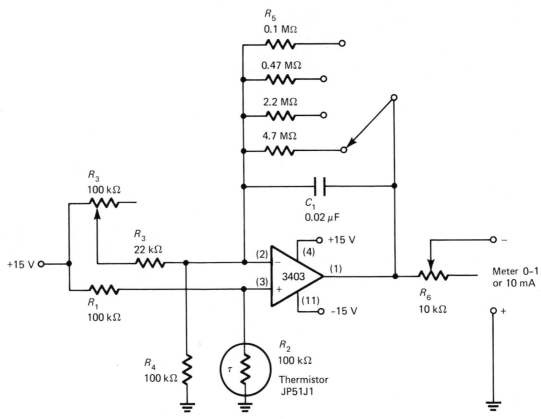

Fig. 18–3. **Wheatstone bridge amplifier with adjustable gain.**

EQUATIONS

$$\frac{R_1}{R_2} = \frac{R_3}{R_4} \qquad (18\text{-}1)$$

$$R_2 = \frac{R_1 R_4}{R_3} \qquad (18\text{-}2)$$

$$G \text{ (stage gain)} = \frac{R_5}{R_3} \qquad (18\text{-}3)$$

MATERIALS REQUIRED

ACTIVE DEVICES
  1 MC3403
RESISTORS: 5%, 14 W
  1 10 kΩ
  1 22 kΩ

3 100 kΩ
1 0.47 mΩ
1 2.2 mΩ
1 4.7 mΩ
1 10-kΩ potentiometer
CAPACITORS: disc, Mylar, electrolytic, 20%, 25 V
  1 0.02 μF
MISCELLANEOUS COMPONENTS:
  1 Socket, 14-pin
  1 Thermistor, 100 kΩ at 25°C
  1 Milliammeter, 0 to 1 mA
TEST INSTRUMENTS:
  Oscilloscope, dual trace, 5-in
  Function generator, 10 Hz to 1 MHz
  Digital multimeter
  Power supply, ±15 V, 50 mA

TESTS AND MEASUREMENTS

1. Construct and test the circuit shown in Fig. 18-3 using the component values shown. Balance R_3 so that the meter reads 0. (NOTE: Set the calibration potentiometer R_6 to midrange initially. This will protect the meter against surges.) Make R_5 equal to 0.47 MΩ. The thermistor, because it is small and fragile, should be mounted in the end of a test probe or other tubing and a filler used, such as epoxy. However, the arrangement shown in Fig. 18-4 will provide satisfactory results.

2. Test the circuit by balancing the output to 0 and checking your skin temperature and the temperature of

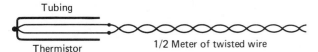

Fig. 18-4. **Thermistor cable assembly.**

your tongue. Try breathing on the thermistor probe. Notice how air currents affect the bridge balance. Adjust R_6 to obtain the amount of deflection desired. Briefly describe your observation.

3. Change R_5 to 4.7 MΩ. Measure the output voltage when temperature is checked again. Does the amplifier saturate or cut off? Is the meter more sensitive with increased amplifier gain?

4. Connect the thermistor leads to an ohmmeter and check the resistance of the thermistor at room temperature. Also check its resistance when the head is placed against your skin. How much change in resistance takes place?

5. Set R_6 to midrange, and set $R_5 = 0.1$ MΩ. Connect the ground ($-$) lead of your voltmeter to pin 2 and the other lead to pin 3. Balance the bridge by adjusting R_3 for zero output. Determine the amount of differential voltage produced by the thermistor when held between your forefinger and thumb.

6. Using the conditions established in step 5, change the DC bridge source to -15 V and explain what differences you observe.

FOR FURTHER RESEARCH

Bridge-type circuits can also be used in AC circuits. Two legs of the bridge are replaced with capacitors whose X_C values take the place of R. Alternating-current bridges are required for certain reactance-type transducers used for the measurement of pressure and flow. Figure 18-5 shows an AC bridge in which resistors R_1 and R_2 are replaced by capacitors. Capacitor C_2 is a known capacitor with minimum dielectric loss (Mylar-suggested), and capacitor C_1 is an unknown or

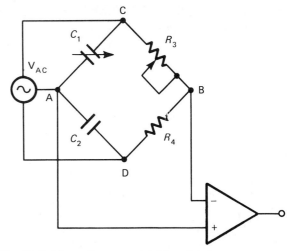

Fig. 18-5. **Alternating-current bridge circuit.**

the capacitance of a transducer whose changes will unbalance the bridge. The equations relating to this bridge are as follows:

1. X_{c_1} (R_1 in original bridge) $= \dfrac{1}{6.28fC_1}$

2. X_{c_1} (R_2 in original bridge) $= \dfrac{1}{6.28fC_2}$

3. $\dfrac{X_{c_1}}{X_{c_2}} = \dfrac{R_3}{R_4}$ or $X_{c_1} = \dfrac{X_{c_2} R_3}{R_4}$

Since $X_C = (1/6.28fC)$, then

$$\frac{1}{6.28fC_1} = \frac{R_3}{R_4} \left(\frac{1}{6.28fC_2} \right)$$

4. Solving for C_1: $C_1 = \dfrac{C_2 R_3}{R_4}$

The sensitivity of the bridge depends on the bridge voltage and the ratio of the unbalanced voltage to unbalanced reactance or resistance (X_{c_1} or R_1).

$$\text{Bridge sensitivity (BS)} = \frac{dAB}{dx_{c_1}} = \frac{-V \text{ (volts)}}{4X_{c_1} \text{ (ohms)}}$$

SELF-TEST

Test your comprehension of the subject by answering the following questions.

1. The advantage of the bridge amplifier is that it provides high _____ and a rugged meter.

2. The highest gain that can be provided by the amplifier shown in Fig. 18-3 is _____.

3. The computed gain (question 2) makes a 1-mA meter appear to be _____ meter.

4. A thermistor has a _____ coefficient of resistance.

5. The output voltage swing of the amplifier in a bridge is limited by the _____ voltage.

SELF-TEST ANSWERS
1. Sensitivity
2. 213
3. Approximately 5 μA
4. Negative
5. Supply

19 PHOTODETECTOR AMPLIFIERS

OBJECTIVES

Upon completion of this experiment, construction of circuitry, testing, and evaluation of data, you will be able to:

1. *Test and evaluate photodetection circuits which use photoconductive cells and operational amplifiers*

2. *Apply photodetection circuits to instrument applications*

DISCUSSION

The circuit shown in Fig. 19-1 uses a high-gain operational amplifier and a photoconductive cell for the detection of light intensities. The amplifier, using ¼ of an MC3403, has a 4.7-MΩ resistor in its feedback. The gain of the amplifier is determined by the ratio of R_1 to R_2. Since the cell's resistance in darkness is very high, there is little gain. When light hits the cell, the cell's resistance is lowered, thus causing an increase in the amplifier gain. The capacitor limits the frequency response and prevents oscillation of the amplifier. A 10-k Ω potentiometer R_4 is arranged in a bridge circuit in order to balance the meter to 0 with no light.

Photoconductive cells with filters can be used to measure infrared (IR), ultraviolet (UV), and normal light. Such arrangements have applications in industry and biomedical electronics.

EQUATIONS

$$G = \frac{R_1}{R_2} \qquad (19\text{-}1)$$

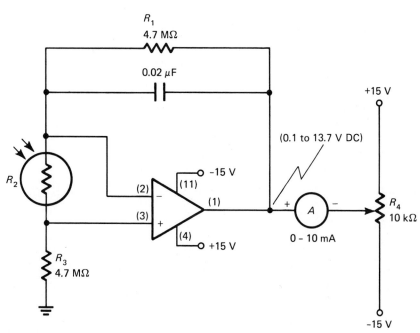

Fig. 19–1. **Photodetector amplifier.**

MATERIALS REQUIRED

ACTIVE DEVICES:
  1 MC3403
RESISTORS: 5%, ¼ W
  2 4.7 MΩ
  1 10-kΩ potentiometer
CAPACITORS: disc, Mylar, electrolytic, 20%, 25 V
  1 0.02 μF

MISCELLANEOUS COMPONENTS:
  1 Socket, 14-pin
  1 Photoresistive cell
TEST INSTRUMENTS:
  Oscilloscope, dual trace, 5 in
  Function generator, 10 Hz to 1 MHz
  Digital multimeter
  Power supply, $+15$ V, 50 mA
  Panel meter, 0 to 10 mA (IRVOM)

TESTS AND MEASUREMENTS

1. Construct the circuit shown in Fig. 19-1 and keep the photoconductive cell covered with black tape or some other black cover. Using a milliammeter with a 10-mA range, adjust the balance potentiometer for a current reading of 0.

2. Measure the output voltage (pin 1) when the cell is dark and light. What is the range the voltage changes?

3. Measure the resistance of the cell with an ohmmeter when the cell is dark and when it is light. Record the resistance under both conditions.

4. Calculate the gain of the amplifier using the resistance measurement in Step 3 when the cell is light.

FOR FURTHER RESEARCH

5. Suppose your light source was a small 5-V lamp whose light output was to remain constant. Variations in materials placed between the lamp and cell causes changes in the cell's resistance. The cell's current is maintained by a constant-current source. Draw a circuit showing the light source whose intensity is held constant and the photodetection circuit.

6. In a medical instrument called the *oximeter*, the light is passed through blood in order to determine the blood-oxygen present. Red and IR cells are used, and both measurements are made simultaneously. Draw a circuit showing two light sources, two cells and amplifiers that you think could be used as a basis for the instrument. The difference between the output in both cells is desired.

SELF-TEST

Test your comprehension of the subject by answering the following questions.

1. The resistance of a photocell _____ when exposed to light.
2. The resistance of a photocell to darkness is in the _____ resistance range.
3. As the resistance of the photocell decreases, the gain of the amplifier _____.
4. If the cell resistance to darkness exceeds 10 MΩ, the output voltage of the amplifier will be near _____.
5. The value of the bleeder current in the balance control is _____.

SELF-TEST ANSWERS
1. Decreases
2. Megohm
3. Increases
4. Zero
5. 3 mA

20 TRANSDUCERS AND SOLID-STATE SWITCHING

OBJECTIVES

Upon completion of this experiment, construction of circuitry, testing, and evaluation of data, you will be able to:

1. *Construct, test, and evaluate multiple transducer control circuitry using linear integrated circuits*

2. *Use electronic switching techniques in conjunction with operational amplifier temperature and light-sensing circuits*

3. *Arrange bridge circuitry for operational amplifier inputs using transducers*

DISCUSSION

Applications for transducers in controlling and detecting are limited virtually by the imagination of the design engineer. Temperature-, light-, and sound-sensing devices are being used extensively in alarm and alerting systems, counting and sorting apparatus, biomedical equipment, and safety and control devices. Such wide use of transducers makes it impossible to address each circuit arrangement individually; however, much of the information herein presented is applicable to all.

Refer to the circuit shown in Fig. 20-1. A temperature-sensing element is used in one leg of a bridge circuit that provides the input to operational amplifier A_1. Any increase in temperature causes the thermistor resistance to decrease and the bridge to become unbalanced. The output voltage of the "disturbed" bridge forces the noninverting input in a positive direction (because of the placement of the thermistor in the bridge) and the output of amplifier A_1 goes high. Similarly, the output of amplifier A_2 goes high when the photocell is exposed to a light source. However, amplifier A_2 functions as an inverting follower.

Transistor Q_1 acts as a switch and, since it is of the NPN variety, it requires a positive potential at the base to cause conduction. This positive voltage is provided when either or both sensing elements become excited. In the on state a potential is developed across the emitter resistor of Q_1. This potential is used to turn on a tone oscillator.

A digital buffer chip (SN7404) is used for the tone generator. An astable oscillator, which consists essentially of two amplifiers, feeds a parallel amplifier arrangement of drivers for the speaker. By supplying or removing the V_{CC} potential, the oscillator is rendered functional. Frequency-determining components are capacitor C_1 and resistor R_{10}.

MATERIALS REQUIRED

ACTIVE DEVICES:
  1 MC3403
  1 SN7404
  1 2N3904 Transistor
RESISTORS: 5%, ¼ W
  1 270 Ω
  2 2.7 kΩ
  1 33 kΩ
  2 100 kΩ
  3 4.7 MΩ
  1 100 kΩ-Potentiometer
CAPACITORS: Disc, Mylar, electrolytic, 20%, 25 V
  1 3 µF
  1 5 µF
  1 100 µF
MISCELLANEOUS COMPONENTS:
  2 Sockets, 14-pin
  1 Thermistor, 100 kΩ
  1 Photoresistive cell
  1 Speaker, 8Ω
TEST INSTRUMENTS:
  Oscilloscope, dual trace, 5 in
  Function Generator, 10 Hz to 1 MHz
  Digital multimeter
  Power supply, ±15 V, 50 mA

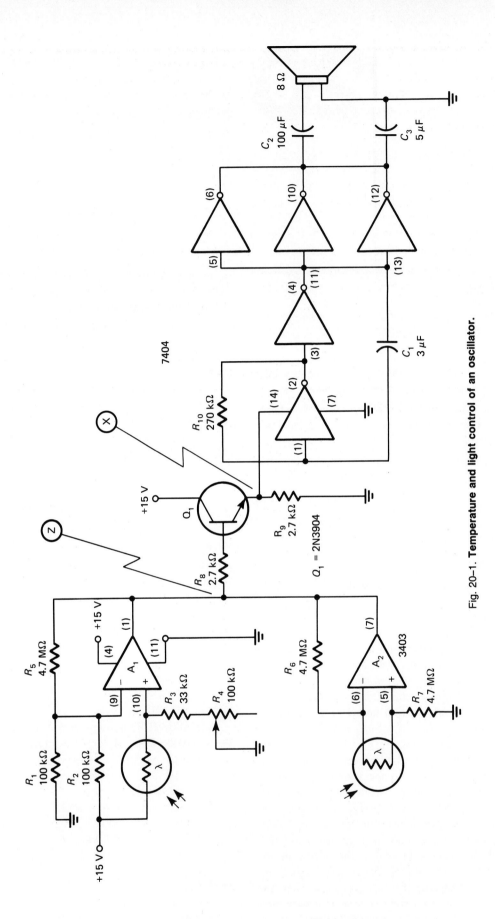

Fig. 20–1. Temperature and light control of an oscillator.

1. Construct the circuit shown in Fig. 20-1 using the component values shown. Measure and record static voltages on the operational amplifiers and transistor.

NOTE: The SN7404 does not have any potential applied until Q_1 is turned on. You are cautioned to balance the thermistor bridge circuit prior to taking static voltage measurements. To balance the input bridge circuit of amplifier A_1, adjust potentiometer R_4 to obtain a zero differential potential between IC pins 9 and 10.

2. Manually heat the thermistor with your hand while observing test points Z and X on a DC-coupled dual-trace oscilloscope. Record the potentials at the test points.

3. What potentials exist at points Z and X when the photocell is exposed to light?

4. Was the tone generator activated in steps 2 and 3 above?

FOR FURTHER RESEARCH

5. State several applications for circuitry similar to that of this experiment.

6. Incorporate into the circuitry a method of liquid-level detection and provide a diagramatic sketch of component arrangement.

SELF-TEST

Test your comprehension of the subject by answering the following questions. Refer to Fig. 20-1.

1. Amplifiers A_1 and A_2 act as a logic _____ circuit.

2. The output voltage of amplifiers A_1 and A_2 go in a _____ direction when either a temperature or light change takes place.

3. The SN7404 is a _____ logic chip.

4. Paralleling the three output amplifiers _____ the power output and _____ _____ the output resistance.

5. The oscillator frequency is determined by _____ and _____.

SELF-TEST ANSWERS
1. OR
2. Positive
3. Hex inverter
4. Increases, lowers
5. C_1 and R_{10}

OBJECTIVES

Upon completion of this experiment, construction of circuitry, testing, and evaluation of data, you will be able to:

1. *Construct and evaluate low-input current amplifiers used for ramp-and-hold circuits*

2. *Evaluate sample-and-hold circuits*

3. *Evaluate a voltage sample and compare it with a new $+V_{in}$ input.*

DISCUSSION

In some instrumentation applications it is necessary to hold a voltage level which represents an event that has taken place. The length of holding varies according to the quality of the capacitor being charged and the input currents of the operational amplifier. Often, low-leakage-current FET switches are used to reduce the drain on the charged capacitor.

In some hold circuits the charged capacitor is located at the input to the operational amplifier, while in others the charged capacitor is part of an integrator circuit (IC). In this experiment the integrator amplifier is used with an amplifier biasing method which reduces the need for the input signal to provide biasing. The result is that the input current is reduced to fractions of a microampere. With the addition of a few components, the sampled voltage can be compared with a new input voltage and adjustments can be made in the holding voltage if it differs from the new input.

Figure 21-1 shows two amplifiers *A* and *B* which are arranged to reduce I_B, biasing current. The input biasing current I_{B1} is supplied by amplifier *B* via resistors R_1, R_2, and R_3 and is used to adjust the effective input current I_{B2} to zero. Since the input signal does not have to provide biasing current for the amplifier, the input looks like a very high impedance and lends itself to "holding" applications. If R_3 were omitted and $R_1 =$

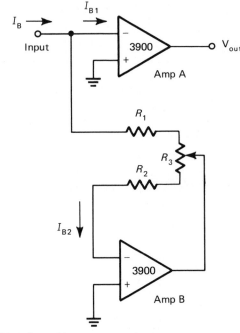

Fig. 21–1. **Input bias current reduction.**

$R_2 = 10$ MΩ, the I_B effective could be reduced to less than $I_B/10$. This may be adequate for some applications.

Figure 21-2 shows the same amplifier arrangement with the addition of an integrating capacitor, C_1, and two inputs. The output is a low-drift ramp-and-hold voltage. The output can be ramped up with a positive input to V_2 or ramped down with a positive input to V_1 (inverting input). Because of the low input current, I_B, the DC output level remains in the hold mode. The output voltage and its slope is a function of either input voltage (V_1 or V_2).

Now refer to the sample and hold section of Fig. 21-3. Two clamping transistors and a third amplifier have been added. The gating voltage is applied to Q_1 and Q_2, and the sample signal voltage is applied to the positive input of amplifier *C*. A positive pulse input to Q_1 and Q_2 turns these two transistors on. The circuitry is in a "hold" mode when the transistors are on. (The collectors go to ground and no signal is applied from amplifier C). When Q_1 and Q_2 are off (no control input pulse), the output $V_{out\ 1}$ will ramp up or down until the output voltage is equal to the DC signal from amplifier C.

Resistor R_7 provides a fixed down ramp which is compared or balanced with amplifier C output via resistor R_5. When transistors Q_1 and Q_2 are off, the feedback loop from amplifier C assures that the output $V_{out\ 1}$ will follow the input signal $(+V_{in})$ to amplifier C. If the input voltage changes, the previous hold voltage is shifted to the value of the new input. Resistor R_3, shown in Figs. 21-1 and 21-2, has been omitted in this circuit. Amplifier B provides biasing to amplifier A. The stored voltage appears at $V_{out\ 1}$, and when V_{in} changes, the continuous comparison between $V_{out\ 1}$ and V_{in} results in change in the sample voltage held by C_1. Capacitor C_1 should not only have low leakage, but should also be nonpolarized. For best results, C_1 should have a Teflon, polyethylene, or polycarbonate dielectric. The sample-and-hold circuitry is evaluated in the "Tests and Measurements" section. The IC selected, LM3900, is a *Norton amplifier* with a typical input bias current of 30 μA. See Appendix A for data on the LM3900. Applications for this type of circuit include control systems and instrumentation.

EQUATIONS

$$V_{out\ 1} = V_{in} \text{ (hold)}$$

where t_1 is greater than t_0 and is less than t_2. (21-1)

$$V_{out\ 1} = A_{out\ 2}\ (V_{in}) \qquad \text{for period } t_1 \text{ to } t_2$$

where $A_{out\ 2}$ is equal to gain of amplifier C. (21-2)

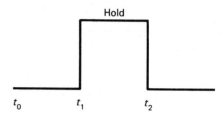

Fig. 21–4. **Timing action of hold circuit.**

MATERIALS REQUIRED

ACTIVE DEVICES:
  1 LM3900
  3 2N3904 Transistor
  1 1N914 Diode
RESISTORS: 5%, 1/4 W
  1 470 Ω
  1 3.3 kΩ
  1 4.7 kΩ
  1 10 kΩ
  1 22 kΩ
  1 33 kΩ
  3 47 kΩ
  2 270 kΩ
  1 150 kΩ
  1 330 kΩ
  1 470 kΩ
  1 1 MΩ
  2 10 MΩ
  1 10 kΩ Potentiometer
  1 100 kΩ Potentiometer
CAPACITORS: disc, Mylar, electrolytic, 20%, 25 V
  1 0.22 μF
MISCELLANEOUS COMPONENTS:
  1 Socket, 14-pin
  3 Sockets, transistor
  1 Switch, SPST
TEST INSTRUMENTS:
  Oscilloscope, dual-trace, 5-in
  Function generator, 10 Hz to 1 MHz
  Digital multimeter
  Power supply, ±15 V, 50 mA
  Resistance decade box

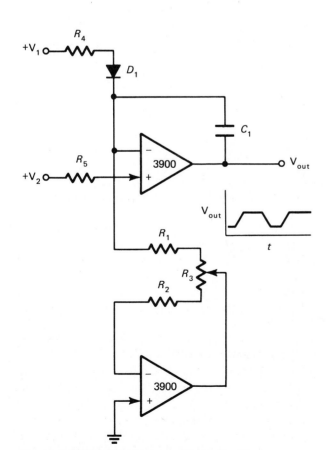

Fig. 21–2. **Diagram of a ramp-and-hold circuit.**

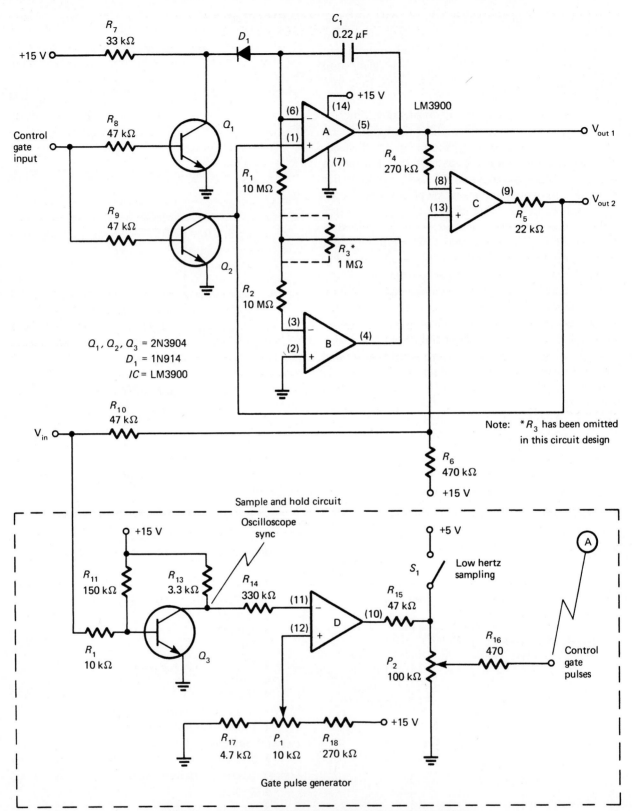

Fig. 21–3. **Sample-and-hold circuit with positive pulse generator.**

NOTE: A positive pulse generator is required. If it is not available, the circuitry enclosed within the dashed lines drawn in Fig. 21-3 can be built and used.

1. Construct the circuit shown in Fig. 21-3 using component values as shown.

2. Without a control pulse input or signal input to V_{in}, measure and record the static voltages (ensuring that V + applied to R_7 is equal to 15 V DC).

NOTE: In the following steps the circuitry of the gate pulse generator shown was used to obtain the positive pulse required for the gate control input. Two controls are provided in the circuitry; potentiometer P_1 allows the pulse width to be varied and potentiometer P_2 controls the pulse amplitude.

3. Ensure that P_1 and P_2 are set to minimum. Apply a sine wave of 100 to 150 mV at 100 Hz to V_{in}. While monitoring $V_{out\ 1}$ on an oscilloscope, adjust V_{in} to the maximum allowable amplitude without distorting $V_{out\ 1}$. Record the values of V_{in} and $V_{out\ 1}$.

4. It is necessary at this point to check the operation of the gate pulse generator. Without disturbing the level of V_{in} established in step 3, measure and record the output waveshape at pin 10 of amplifier D (make sure that P_1 is set to the minimum resistance).

5. Since the width of the gating pulse determines the hold time, determine the range of pulse widths obtainable with P_1 while observing the pulse at pin 10 of amplifier D.

6. Measure and record the output waveshape observed at test point A with P_2 adjusted to maximum. (NOTE: For this measurement, it is necessary to totally isolate the test point from the sample-and-hold circuitry.) Set P_1 to minimum.

Up to this point we have been concerned with biasing and signal levels. If the results obtained in these tests and measurements were favorable, the remaining steps will evaluate sample and hold.

7. Using a dual-trace oscilloscope, connect channel A to view V_{in} and channel B to observe $V_{out\ 1}$. Set P_1 and P_2 of the gate pulse generator to minimum. Feed V_{in} with a 300-mV, volt, 100-Hz sine wave and ensure that $V_{out\ 1}$ is not distorted. Is V_{in} in phase with $V_{out\ 1}$? Explain.

8. Now move the channel A probe from V_{in} to the control gate input while maintaining all other conditions of step 7. Determine the level of pulse required to set Q_1 and Q_2 to an on state. Provide a sketch of the pattern observed on channel B. (NOTE: It is important that Q_1 and Q_2 be *solidly* biased on). Determine the hold time.

9. Vary P_1 and explain what happens to $V_{out\ 1}$.

SELF-TEST

Test your comprehension of the subject by answering the following questions. Refer to Fig. 21-3.

1. In Fig. 21-3, amplifier A is an _____ circuit.
2. Amplifier D is a _____ circuit.
3. Closing switch S_1 causes the output signal to be _____ level shifted.
4. Amplifier B is connected as a _____ voltage follower.
5. The potentiometer P_1 determines the _____ .

SELF-TEST ANSWERS
1. Integrator
2. Comparator
3. DC
4. Constant
5. Pulse width

22 CAPACITANCE MULTIPLIERS

OBJECTIVES

Upon completion of this experiment, construction of circuitry, testing, and evaluation of data, you will be able to:

1. *Compute and construct an integrated circuit amplifier circuit whose characteristics simulate those of a large capacitor*

2. *Use the simulated capacitor in test circuits*

DISCUSSION

At times it is necessary to eliminate large capacitors from circuits or systems because of their physical bulk. In such instances, a solid-state circuit which simulates a large conventional capacitor can be employed. Thus an understanding of the integrated circuit (IC) capacitance multiplier becomes extremely valuable.

Refer to the circuit shown in Fig. 22-1. A variable-capacitance multiplier is presented. Two sections of the 3403 are used; section *A* acts as a follower to isolate the loading effect created by R_S *(series resistance of the multiplied capacitance), and section B* functions as the multiplier. Circuit performance is described by Eq.

(22-1) and (22-2). Because the series resistance is so high, the Q of the multiplied capacitance suffers. Thus the circuit is not used in filter or tuned circuit applications; however, it is widely applied in servo compensation networks and timing circuits.

EQUATIONS

$$C_T = C_1 \left(1 + \frac{R_B}{R_S} \right) \qquad (22\text{-}1)$$

$$C = \frac{1}{6.28 f X_C} \qquad (22\text{-}2)$$

MATERIALS REQUIRED

ACTIVE DEVICES:
  1 MC3403
RESISTORS: 5%, 1/4 W
  1 1.5 kΩ
  1 2.2 kΩ
  1 10 kΩ Potentiometer
CAPACITORS: disc, Mylar, electrolytic, 20%, 25 V
  1 47 pF

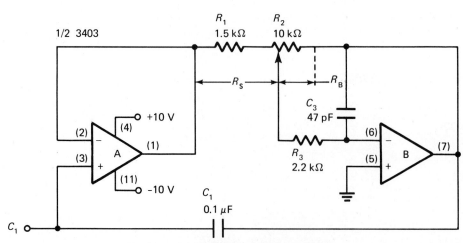

Fig. 22–1. **Capacitance multiplying circuit.**

1 0.1 μF			
1 100 μF			

1 0.1 μF
1 100 μF
MISCELLANEOUS COMPONENTS:
   1 Socket, 14-pin
TEST INSTRUMENTS:

Oscilloscope, dual-trace, 5-in
Function generator, 10 Hz to 1 MHz
Digital multimeter
Power supply, ±15 V, 50 mA
Capacitance decade box

TESTS AND MEASUREMENTS

1. Compute the maximum and minimum values of C_T for the circuit illustrated in Fig. 22-1 using the component values shown.

2. Using the test circuit shown in Fig. 22-2, determine the *multiplied capacitance* (C_T). Construct the test circuit. Apply a 2-V p-p sine wave at 100 Hz through variable resistance R_x as shown. Using a dual-trace oscilloscope, monitor V_1 on channel A and V_3 on channel B. Vary R_x to set $V_3 = 0.7V_1$ (at this point the V_2 rms voltage will equal the V_3 rms voltage). Use a digital voltmeter (DVM) or vacuum-tube voltmeter (VTVM) to compare the rms values of V_3 and V_2 and readjust R_x if necessary to obtain V_3 (rms) = V_2 (rms). Measure and record the voltage and resistance values required to complete Table 22-1 with R_2 set at maximum (minimum capacitance) (rms = root mean square).

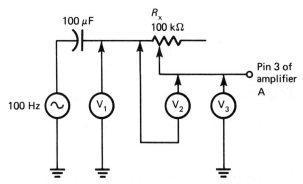

Fig. 22–2. **Test circuit for determining capacitance value.**

the equation, determine the measured value of C_T.

4. Ignoring the series resistance of the multiplied capacitance, use the value of R_x to determine C_T.

5. Using the procedure outlined in step 2 above, set R_2 to minimum (maximum capacitance) and determine the measured values of C_T per steps 3 and 4 above.

6. Compare the measured and computed values of C_T.

TABLE 22-1

	Volts rms	Volts p-p		
V_1			R_b	
V_2		———	R_s	
V_3			R_x	

3. Substituting the measured values of R_B and R_S into

SELF-TEST

Test your comprehension of the subject by answering the following questions.

1. In Fig. 22-1 amplifier A is a _____ follower circuit.
2. In Fig. 22-1 amplifier B is an _____ circuit.
3. If $R_B = 10k\Omega$ and $R_S = 1.5k\Omega$, what is the equivalent capacitance?
4. The capacitance multiplier has a _____ Q.
5. The capacitance multiplier is designed only for high frequency applications (true or false).

SELF-TEST ANSWERS
1. Voltage
2. Integrator
3. 84 μF
4. Low
5. False

EXPERIMENT 23 SIMULATED INDUCTORS

OBJECTIVES

Upon completion of this experiment, construction of circuitry, testing, and evaluation of data, you will be able to:

1. *Compute and construct an integrated circuit amplifier circuit whose characteristics simulate those of an inductor*
2. *Use the simulated inductor in test circuits*
3. *Identify simulated inductor circuits whose terminals are above ground*

DISCUSSION

Circuits such as filters, oscillators, and amplifiers often require the use of inductors. Inductors often are bulky and present mechanical problems, and designers look for ways of using *RC* circuits to replace them. In this experiment an operational amplifier is used to simulate an inductor. Figure 23-1 shows the basic circuit and its equivalent circuit.

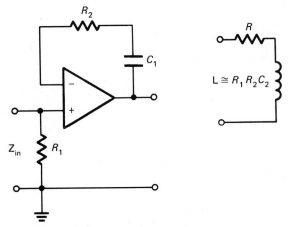

Fig. 23–1. **Circuit for simulating inductance.**

The input impedance Z_{in} and the Q of the circuit are dependent on the component values selected.

$$Z = \frac{R_1 J\omega_0 R_1 R_2 C_1}{J\omega_0 C_1 (R_1 + R_2 - AR_1) + 1}$$

When $(R_1/R_2) = (1/A - 1)$, the above equation reduces to

$$Z_{in} = R_1 + j\omega_0 R_1 R_2 C_1$$

since $j\omega_0 C_1 (R_1 + R_2 - AR_1)$ becomes zero.

The resultant equation represents an inductor and resistor in series. The value of Q is increased by reducing the value of R_1.

EQUATIONS

$$L \cong R_1 R_2 C_1 \qquad (23\text{-}1)$$

$$Z_{in} = R_1 + j\omega_0 R_1 R_2 C_1 \qquad (23\text{-}2)$$

$$X_L = 6.28 \, fL \qquad (23\text{-}3)$$

MATERIALS REQUIRED

ACTIVE DEVICES:
 1 MC3403
RESISTORS: 5%, 1/4 W
 1 100 Ω
 1 4.7 kΩ
 4 22 kΩ
 2 2.2 MΩ
 1 10 MΩ
CAPACITORS: disc, Mylar, electrolytic, 20%, 25 V
 1 0.01 μF
 1 0.1 μF
 1 0.47 μF
 1 1 μF
MISCELLANEOUS COMPONENTS:
 1 Socket, 14-pin

TEST INSTRUMENTS:

   Oscilloscope, dual-trace, 5-in
   Function generator, 10 Hz to 1 MHz

Digital multimeter
Power supply, ± 15 V, 50 mA
Capacitance decade box

TESTS AND MEASUREMENTS

1. Construct the circuit shown in Fig. 23-2 using the component values indicated. Measure and record static voltages.

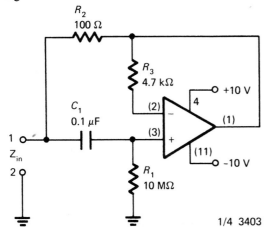

Fig. 23-2. **Test circuit for simulated inductor.**

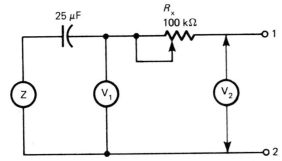

Fig. 23-3. **Substitution method for measuring inductance.**

2. Compute the inductance value using Eq. (23-1).

3. Connect the test circuit shown in Fig. 23-3 to the circuit shown in Fig. 23-2. Use a 2-V p-p sine wave and set $V_2 = 0.7V_1$ by varying R_x. Remove R_x from the circuit and measure and record its value; this value of $R_x = X_L$. Determine the value of L. (NOTE: A dual-trace oscilloscope, DVM, or VTVM may be used to measure the generator and input signal voltage.)

4. Compare the results obtained in steps 2 and 3 above.

5. Repeat steps 2 and 3 substituting a 0.47-μF capacitor for C_1 at 20 Hz. Do the computed and measured values come within 10 percent of one another?

6. Change C_1 to a 0.01-μF capacitor and repeat steps 2 and 3 at 1 kHz. What is the percent difference between the computed and measured values of L?

FOR FURTHER RESEARCH

A shortcoming of the circuit of Fig. 23-2 is that one terminal is at ground. In audio- and power-supply filter circuits both inductor terminals must be above ground. The circuit presented in Fig. 23-4 provides for "floating" terminals. This circuit is an amplifier–gyrator-simulated inductor that provides for operation with both terminals above ground. For the component values shown in Fig. 23-4, the circuit will appear as an inductance ranging in the thousands of henries at audio frequencies.

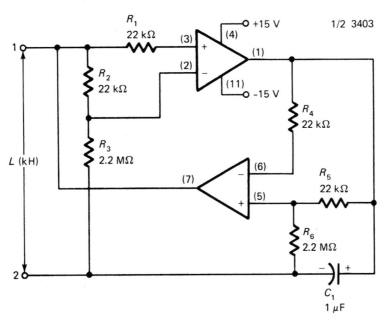

Fig. 23-4. **Inductor circuit with floating terminals.**

Test your comprehension of the subject by answering the following questions.

1. The input impedance in a simulated inductor is greater than its input _____
2. In a tuned circuit containing L, C, and R components, the Q of the circuit is determined mainly by _____.
3. If R_1, R_2, and C_1 equal 1 MΩ, 500 Ω, and 0.05 μF, respectively, what is the equivalent inductance?
4. While the inductance in a simulated inductor circuit may be high, its Q is _____.

SELF-TEST ANSWERS
1. Resistance
2. L, R
3. 25 H
4. Low

24 TIMER/MONOSTABLE OSCILLATORS

OBJECTIVES

Upon completion of this study, construction of circuitry, testing, and evaluation of data, you will be able to:

1. *Construct and test timer circuits which use specially designed integrated circuits*

2. *Modify circuitry in order to obtain desired time delay*

3. *Apply timer circuitry to practical problems*

DISCUSSION

The timer shown in Fig. 24-1 is designed and constructed using a versatile integrated circuit, the LM556 (a dual LM555). Two timers are built on one chip. They are independent and will work separately. (For technical data, see Appendix A.) The timing function is provided by resistor R_A in conjunction with capacitor C_1.

The circuit is a monostable (single-state) oscillator. When a negative-going pulse of less than V_{CC} is fed to the trigger input, the temporary internal short across the capacitor is released and the output of the IC is shifted to a high state. The capacitor charges exponentially for a period of $t = 1.1 R_A C_1$, at the end of which time the voltage equals $2/3\ V_{CC}$. The internal voltage comparator then resets the flip-flop, which, in turn, discharges the capacitor and drives the output to its original low state. During the timing period additional triggers will not affect the timing. The timer can be reset at any time, however, by applying a negative-going pulse to the reset input. The timer will remain in the low state until the next negative trigger arrives.

The IC also has many other applications, including frequency modulation, frequency division, and wave generation.

EQUATIONS

$$t = 1.1 R_A C_1 \qquad (24\text{-}1)$$

MATERIALS REQUIRED

ACTIVE DEVICES:
  1 LM556
RESISTORS: 5%, 1/4 W
  1 100-kΩ Potentiometer
CAPACITORS: disc, Mylar, electrolytic, 20%, 25 V
  1 25 μF
  1 0.01 μF
MISCELLANEOUS COMPONENTS:
  1 Socket, 14-pin
  1 Switch, SPST
TEST INSTRUMENTS:
  Oscilloscope, dual-trace, 5-in
  Function generator, 10 Hz to 1 MHz
  Digital multimeter
  Power supply, $\pm$15 V, 50 mA

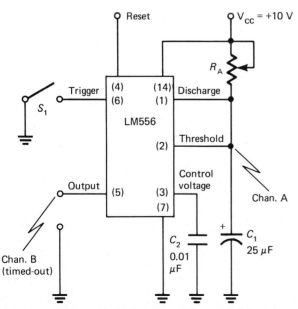

Fig. 24–1. **Timing and monostable oscillator circuit diagram.**

1. Construct the circuit as shown in Fig. 24-1 using a 25-μF capacitor for C_1 and a 100-kΩ potentiometer for R_A. Connect channel A (DC coupled) of a dual-trace oscilloscope to the output (pin 5) and channel B (DC coupled) to pin 2. This arrangement will permit you to observe the capacitor charging and the output level as it shifts (timed-out).

2. Trigger the circuit by momentarily grounding pin 6 and observe both pins 5 and 2 on your oscilloscope. Does the output shift to the high state? By how many volts does the output level shift?

3. How long is the time period between triggering and the output's return to the low state with $R_A = 50$ kΩ?

4. Does the time period follow the stated equation?

5. Compute the component values necessary for time-out periods of 5s and 10s.

6. Construct the 5-s timer and, after triggering, try to retrigger. What happens? Try touching the reset to ground after 1 to 2 s. What happens to the output?

FOR FURTHER RESEARCH

7. Redraw the circuit schematic and add an LED (light-emitting diode) indicator which will display when the timer is in the timed-out state.

8. Insert the components needed to add the LED indicator. Does the additional circuitry work?

SELF-TEST

Test your comprehension of the subject by answering the following questions.

1. Once the monostable time has started, it can be stopped by a trigger pulse (true or false).
2. If a 10-V power supply is used, a positive-going trigger pulse of 3 V is required (true or false).
3. The output pulse or the timer is _____-going.
4. The trigger pulse must be _____-going.
5. If $R_A = 2.2$ MΩ and $C_1 = 100$ μF, the timed period, after triggering, is _____.

SELF-TEST ANSWERS
1. False
2. False (negative pulse)
3. Positive
4. Negative
5. 4 min

25 LINEAR CAPACITANCE METERS

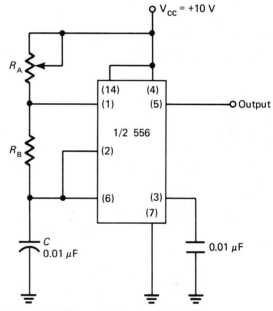

Fig. 25–1. **Astable oscillator circuit diagram.**

OBJECTIVES

Upon completion of this experiment, construction of circuitry, testing, and data evaluation, you will be able to:

1. *Design and build an astable multivibrator circuit using a special integrated circuit model LM556*
2. *Compute component values to establish periods of the timer cycle*
3. *Apply an astable oscillator circuit to the design of an instrument for measuring the capacitance of a capacitor*

DISCUSSION

In the circuit shown in Fig. 25-1 two resistors, R_A and R_B, are used to set the timing of the circuit for the high state. When capacitor C_1 reaches 2/3 V_{cc}, it is discharged through resistor R_B. Figure 25-2 shows the output waveform. Thus $R_A + R_B$ can be used to set the time t_1, and resistor R_B can be used to set the time t_2. The equations provided will enable you to design an astable oscillator whose time periods can be easily established.

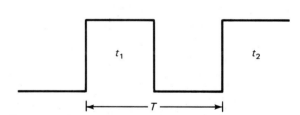

Fig. 25–2. **Timed period of an astable oscillator.**

EQUATIONS

$$t_1 \text{ (high)} = 0.693(R_A + R_B)C \qquad (25\text{-}1)$$

$$t_2 \text{ (low)} = 0.693(R_B)C \qquad (25\text{-}2)$$

$$T = t_1 + t_2 = 0.693(R_A + 2R_B)C \qquad (25\text{-}3)$$

$$f_0 \text{ (frequency of oscillation)} = \frac{1.44}{(R_A + 2R_B)C} = \frac{1}{T}$$

$$(25\text{-}4)$$

MATERIALS REQUIRED

ACTIVE DEVICES:
  1 LM556
RESISTORS: 5%, 1/4 W
  Assorted resistance values
  1 100-kΩ Potentiometer
CAPACITORS: disc, Mylar, electrolytic, 20%, 25 V
  2 0.01 μF
MISCELLANEOUS COMPONENTS:
  1 Socket, 14-pin

Oscilloscope, dual-trace, 5-in
Function generator, 10 Hz to 1 MHz
Digital multimeter

Power supply, $\pm$ 15 V, 50 mA
Resistance decade box

TESTS AND MEASUREMENTS

1. Determine the values of R_A and R_B for a 10-ms period *(T)* where t_1 is 7 ms. Use a capacitor value of 0.01 μF.

2. Using the computed values and a 0.01-μF capacitor, construct the circuit shown in Fig. 25-1. Before connecting the positive voltage to the IC, set the supply voltage to 10 V. (NOTE: the chip has a maximum voltage of 18 V).

3. Measure the time periods t_1 and t_2 on your oscilloscope and determine whether the periods measured follow the computed values.

4. How much output voltage is available when $V_{CC} = +10$ V?

5. Parallel your resistor R_B with a resistance decade box set to 10 MΩ. Reduce the decade setting while watching the waveshape on the oscilloscope. Which time period is changing, t_1 or t_2?

6. Lower the supply voltage to 5 V. Does the frequency change with a change of supply voltage?

most to zero through diode D_1. Since the charge Q on the capacitor is equal to $C_x V$, the effective current through the meter equals

$$I_{eff} = C_x Vf$$

where C_x is the unknown capacity, V (V_{CC}) is the charging voltage, and f is the frequency of the charging voltage. For $V_{CC} = 10$ V, Table 25-1 shows the full-scale capacitance range plotted against frequency for a 100-μA ammeter. (Most VOM multimeters have a 100-μA scale.) The 10-kΩ and 4.7-kΩ resistors and 100-μF capacitor reduce the pulses to near DC, thus reducing the pulsations of the meter. Since the unknown capacitor is charged to 10 V, polarity should be observed.

TABLE 25-1

Full-scale Capacity (C_x), in μF	Frequency
100.000 μF	100 kHz
0.001 μF	10 kHz
0.01 μF	1 kHz
0.1 μF	100 Hz
1.0 μF	10 Hz
10.000 μF	1 Hz

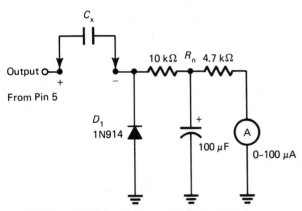

Fig. 25–3. **Circuit diagram for measuring unknown capacitance.**

Capacitance Meter

7. Set the frequency of oscillation to 100 Hz such that $t_1 = 7$ms and $t_2 = 3$ ms.

8. Add the circuit shown in Fig. 25-3 to your output.

Capacitance Meter Operation

When the output square wave is high, the unknown capacitor C_x charges almost to V_{CC} with the current passing through the 100-μA ammeter circuit. When the square wave goes low, the capacitor discharges al-

9. Insert a 0.1-μF capacitor for C_x before turning on your power supply. Turn on your power supply and see if you get a full-scale deflection. How much deflection do you get?
(NOTE: The amount of deflection depends on the meter resistance. If you don't obtain full-scale deflection, use the alternate procedure outlined below for making measurements.)

10. Insert a 0.05-μF capacitor for C_x. How much deflection is obtained?

FOR FURTHER RESEARCH

11. Redesign the timer circuit values of R_A and R_B so that a full-scale deflection of 100 μA translates to 100 pF. Maintain t_1 at a value approximately equal to $2t_2$. Check some capacitors between 10 pF and 100 pF on a capacitance bridge and compare the results with those obtained using the redesigned circuit.

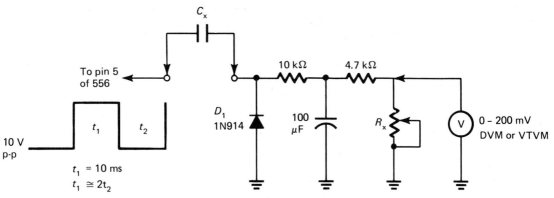

Fig. 25–4. **Direct meter reading of capacitance.**

Alternate Meter Circuit

12. Using the circuit shown in Fig. 25-4, insert a validated 0.1-μF capacitor for C_x (must have been checked on capacitance bridge). Adjust R_x until the DVM reads 100 mV. The meter circuit is now calibrated such that the scale reading translates directly to the value of capacitance.

NOTE: Potentiometer R_x should be approximately 1k Ω to 1.1 kΩ when the meter circuit is correctly calibrated.)

SELF-TEST

Test your comprehension of the subject by answering the following questions.

1. An astable oscillator requires triggering to start (true or false).
2. In an astable oscillator circuit the high time is always equal to the low time (true-false).
3. A timer circuit uses an R value of 100kΩ $(R_A + R_B)$ and a capacitance of 0.001 μF. What is the high time period?
4. If the R_B value of question 3 has a value of 22kΩ, what is the low time period?
5. What is the time period if $R_A = 78$ kΩ, $R_B = 22$ kΩ, and $C = 0.001\mu$F?

SELF-TEST ANSWERS
1. False
2. False
3. 69.3 μs
4. 15.2 μs
5. 84.5 μs

26 TIME-DELAY RELAY CONTROL

OBJECTIVES

Upon completion of this experiment, construction of circuitry, testing, and evaluation of data, you will be able to:

1. *Use the LM556 dual timer for designing and evaluating short and long time-delay relay circuits*
2. *Use the dual-timer chip for sequential timing circuits*
3. *Apply timer circuits to instrumentation problems*

DISCUSSION

The LM556 dual timer IC basically consists of a flip-flop and two comparators which control the charge and discharge of an external capacitor. In this experiment the IC will be utilized for driving a relay. A single timer and a dual timer, operating in sequential action, are used in this laboratory experiment.

Single Timer

The timing period is determined by

$$t_1 = 1.1 R_1 C_1$$

The timer operates as a monostable oscillator. When the timer is not triggered, its capacitor is short-circuited by an internal transistor. When triggered by a negative-going pulse of less than $1/3$ V_{CC}, the short is removed and the capacitor charges until it reaches $2/3$ V_{CC}, at which time the flip-flop recycles and the time period is completed. With high-quality polycarbonate dielectric capacitors, long time delays can be achieved. Additional trigger pulses do not affect the timed period during the charging period. A reset terminal can be used at any time to stop the timing period and recycle the capacitor to 0.

Sequential Timing

Since the LM556 is a dual timer, one section can be used to trigger the second section so the total time is

$$T = t_1 + t_2 = 1.1\ R_1 C_1 + 1.1\ R_2 C_2$$

The two timers are connected by a 0.01-μF capacitor, and the starting pulse is obtained by momentarily shorting the trigger input to ground.

Two circuits are provided for evaluation. One circuit is typical of the single timer. The period of the circuit is a function of $P_1 R_1 C_1$. The other circuit is the sequential timer, with its period established by components $R_7 C_2$.

EQUATIONS

$$t = 1.1\ R_1 C_1$$
$$\text{where } R_1 = P_1 + R_1. \qquad (26\text{-}1)$$

$$T = t_1 + t_2 = 1.1\ R_1 C_1 + 1.1\ R_2 C_2$$
$$\text{where } R_1 = P_1 + R_1. \qquad (26\text{-}2)$$

MATERIALS REQUIRED

ACTIVE DEVICES:
  1 LM556
  1 1.7-V Light-emitting diode (LED)
  1 1N914 Diode
RESISTORS: 5%, 1/4 W
  1 1.5 kΩ
  1 2.7 kΩ
  2 4.7 kΩ
  2 10 kΩ
  1 470 kΩ
  1 47 mΩ
  1 10-kΩ Potentiometer
  1 1-mΩ Potentiometer
CAPACITORS: disc, Mylar, electrolytic, 20%, 25 V
  1 0.01 μF
  1 0.22 μF

1 μF
1 10 μF
MISCELLANEOUS COMPONENTS:
   1 Socket, 14-pin
   1 Relay, 6 to 12 V, 3PST
   2 Switches, SPST

TEST INSTRUMENTS:
   Oscilloscope, dual-trace, 5-in
   Function generator, 10 Hz to 1 MHz
   Digital multimeter
   Power supply, $\pm$15 V, 50 mA

TESTS AND MEASUREMENTS

1. Construct the circuit in Fig. 26-1 using component values as shown and using a V_{CC} of +10 V.

2. Set P_1 for maximum resistance and adjust P_2 so as to obtain maximum time delay. An LED connected to one set of relay contacts will indicate relay lock up. A scope connected through a 4.7-MΩ resistor to pin 1 or pin 2 will permit you to observe the charging time.

3. What is the maximum and minimum time delay obtainable?

4. What effect does P_2 have on the charging voltage?

5. Will the reset switch stop the timing action during the charging period?

Sequential Timer

NOTE: Make all tests and measurements with P_1 at *maximum* resistance.

6. Construct the circuit shown in Fig. 26-2 using component values as shown.

7. Compute the time period for the second half (period t_2) of the timer.

8. Measure the time period for R_7C_2 and compare the computed value from step 2 with the measured value. Explain any difference between the two values.

9. What type of pulse is available at output 1 for triggering of the second section (pin 5)?

10. What is the maximum period $(t_1 + t_2)$ available if both timers are used?

11. Does the reset function during the first or second time period?

12. What is the function of D_1 the relay diode?

FOR FURTHER RESEARCH

13. Design a timer to be used for controlling two functions. At the end of 1 min, close one relay, thus starting a motor. One hour after the motor starts, stop it. Light-emitting diodes will provide visual indications of activated relays.

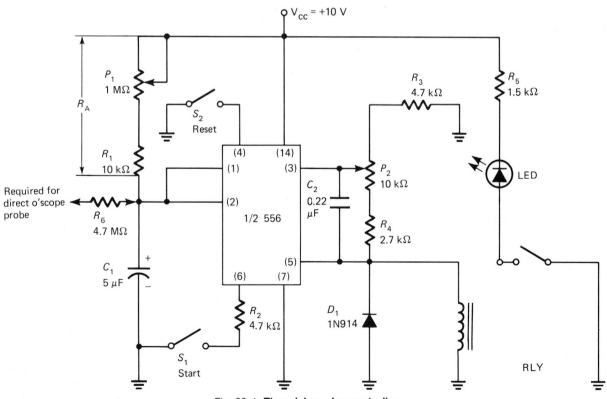

Fig. 26–1. **Time-delay relay controller.**

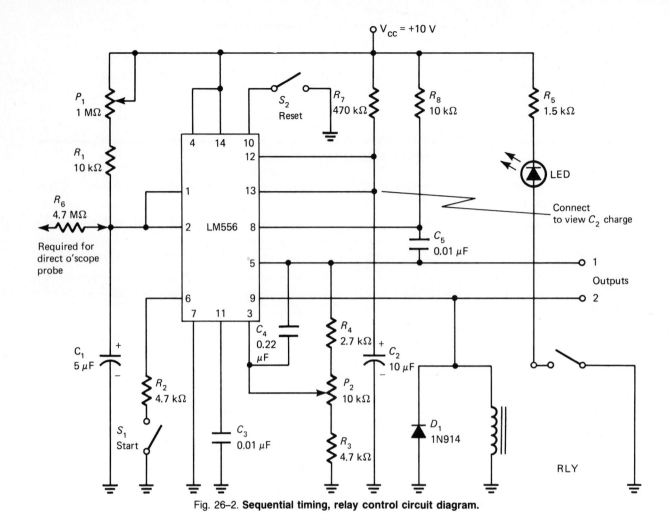

Fig. 26–2. **Sequential timing, relay control circuit diagram.**

SELF-TEST

Test your comprehension of the subject by answering the following questions.

1. What part of the wave from the output at pin 5 is used to trigger the second timer?
2. What is the maximum computed time-out period of the second timer?
3. What does the reset switch do?
4. Diode D_1 is used to eliminate _____ spikes from the relay.
5. The 4.7-MΩ resistor for connection to a scope is needed since the scope's cable will _____ the circuit.

SELF-TEST ANSWERS
1. Negative swing
2. 5.17
3. Stops timing period
4. Negative
5. Load

1. What are the advantages of a differential amplifier as compared to a single-ended amplifier?
2. Define "CMR" and "CMRR."
3. List several applications for differential amplifiers.
4. Will a differential amplifier reject 60-Hz pickup?
5. Why are high-input impedance amplifiers necessary?
6. Why is a constant-voltage source better than a resistor-voltage divider circuit for maintaining a reference voltage?
7. In a constant-voltage source circuit, is the amplifier a voltage follower or voltage amplifier?
8. In a constant-current source circuit, does the load resistor affect the current flow?
9. What is the difference between a "summing" and a "subtracting" circuit?
10. What type of output waveshape is produced by a comparator?
11. What determines the signal trip-voltage level in a comparator?
12. In an integration circuit, what would be the effect of using a "lossy" capacitor for integration?
13. What output waveshape is produced when a square wave is integrated?
14. If an integrator has a long time constant, what type of output would you expect if you integrated 6-V positive peak pulses of 120 Hz?
15. If you differentiate positive-going square-wave pulses, what type of output would you obtain?
16. If the input signal voltages to a multiplier chip exceeds the limit, what can be done in order to obtain a product of the signals?
17. What mathematical functions can be performed by an MC1495 chip?
18. It is desired to use a DC milliammeter to monitor a 1.0-V sine wave output of an audio generator. Could a bridge rectifier of IN914 or a similar diode be used to obtain the DC for the meter?
19. If a 0.5-V AC sine wave signal is fed into a full-wave AC-to-DC converter, what DC voltage output would you expect to obtain?
20. Do thermistors have a negative or positive temperature coefficient?
21. List some factors to be considered in designing a bridge amplifier for temperature measurement.
22. Do photoresistive cells have a negative or a positive coefficient with light?
23. What factors have to be considered in designing a sample-and-hold circuit?
24. List some applications for capacitance and inductance multipliers.
25. List some advantages in using the LM556 chip as a timer or monostable oscillator.

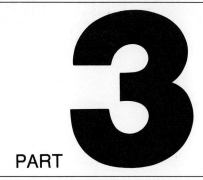

PART **3**

Biomedical
Instrumentation

27 ELECTRO-CARDIOGRAM SIMULATORS

OBJECTIVES

Upon completion of this experiment, construction of circuitry, testing, and evaluation of data, you will be able to:

1. *Design a pulse generator which can be used as an electrocardiogram (ECG or EKG) simulator source*
2. *Provide pulse circuitry with low-level signals*
3. *Using unijunction transistors and operational amplifiers, test and troubleshoot pulse circuitry*

DISCUSSION

In the circuitry for this experiment, a unijunction transistor is used as an oscillator, and operational amplifiers are used as phase inverters in order to provide a differential output signal. Although a linear IC could have been used for the oscillator, the unijunction circuitry is simple and economical. In the oscillator circuit (see Fig. 27-1) the variable resistor P_1 and capacitor C_1 set the frequency of oscillation. Capacitor C_2 and resistor R_4 form a power-supply filter to keep the pulses out of the power supply. Capacitors C_4 and C_6 bypass the high frequencies and roll off the pulse peaks. Capacitor C_3 and potentiometer P_2 are the output of the oscillator circuit. Resistors R_{11}–R_{13} and R_{14}–R_{16} are voltage-divider networks for providing multiple output levels which are adjusted by P_2. The output at $V_{\text{out }1}$ is a positive-going pulse, and the output at $V_{\text{out }2}$ is a negative-going pulse.

EQUATIONS

$$T = RC \qquad (27\text{-}1)$$

$$\text{Operational amplifier gain} = \frac{R_f}{R_{\text{in}}} \qquad (27\text{-}2)$$

$$\text{Beats per minute (bpm)} = \frac{1}{T} \times 60$$
where T is in seconds. $\qquad (27\text{-}3)$

MATERIALS REQUIRED

ACTIVE DEVICES:
   1 MC3403
   1 2N4871 Transistor
RESISTORS: 5%, 1/4 W
   1 270 Ω
   1 180 kΩ
   1 330 Ω
   4 470 Ω
   1 1 kΩ
   3 4.7 kΩ
   3 10 kΩ
   2 100 kΩ
   1 10-kΩ Potentiometer
   1 100-kΩ Potentiometer
CAPACITORS: disc, Mylar, electrolytic, 20%, 25 V
   2 0.05 μF
   1 4.7 μF, Tantalum
   3 5 μF
MISCELLANEOUS COMPONENTS:
   1 Socket, 14-pin
   1 Socket transistor
TEST INSTRUMENTS
   Oscilloscope, dual-trace, 5-in
   Function Generator, 10 Hz to 1 MHz
   Digital Multimeter
   Power Supply, ±15 V, 50 mA

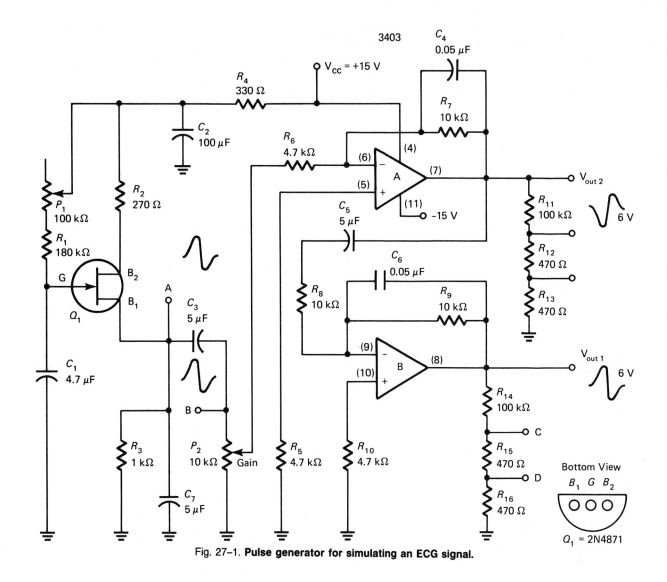

Fig. 27–1. **Pulse generator for simulating an ECG signal.**

TESTS AND MEASUREMENTS

1. Construct the circuit shown in Fig. 27-1 and start by recording the waveshape and measuring the pulse voltage at point A. The pulse should be positive.

2. Measure the voltage and record the waveshape at point B and pin 8 of the IC. Be careful to note any overshoot.

3. Resistors R_{14}–R_{16} form a voltage divider. Monitor the output $V_{out\,1}$ on an oscilloscope and adjust P_2 so as to obtain 1 V. What is the voltage at points C and D when $V_{out\,1}$ equals 1 V?

4. Amplifiers A and B are inverting amplifiers. The gains of the amplifiers are set by

$$\frac{R_7}{R_6} \quad \text{and} \quad \frac{R_9}{R_8},$$

respectively. How do the inputs to R_6 and R_8 compare with $V_{out\,2}$ and $V_{out\,1}$?

5. Determine the value of R_1 for establishing a pulse rate of 60 bpm.

6. Determine the effects of the filter R_2C_2 by comparing the pulse amplitude on C_2 with the $+15$-V line.

FOR FURTHER RESEARCH

7. Design an ECG simulator whose output will produce $\pm 50\ \mu V$ to ± 2-mV pulses with a frequency range selectable in steps of 50, 100, 150, and 200 bpm.

Test your comprehension of the subject by answering the following questions.

1. The pulse pattern on an oscilloscope indicates 0.5 seconds between pulses. How many beats per minute does this represent?
2. A signal of 1 V is to be lowered to microvolts. State an equation for voltage division by two resistors.
3. What is the gain of amplifiers A and B in Fig. 27-1?
4. Why was a tantalytic capacitor used for C_1 in Fig. 27-1?
5. The signal output level at point D in Fig. 27-1 is equal to _____ the output level of C.

SELF-TEST ANSWERS
1. 120
2. $V_{out} = V_{in} = \dfrac{R_2}{(R_1 + R_2)}$

3. $A = 2.1$, $B = 1$
4. To reduce leakage
5. One-half

28 50-HZ or 60-HZ DUAL-NOTCH FILTERS

OBJECTIVES

Upon completion of this experiment, construction of circuitry, testing, and evaluation of data, you will be able to:

1. *Design and construct single- or dual-notch filters for filtering 50-Hz or 60-Hz line frequencies*

2. *Apply notch filter circuitry to differential amplifiers*

3. *Evaluate the characteristics of notch filters used for power-line filtering.*

DISCUSSION

Power-line magnetic fields and their induced voltages cause disturbing patterns in ECG, electroencephalogram (EEG), and electromyogram (EMG), tachometers and many other types of biomedical instrumentation. Since a typical biomedical amplifier usually has a frequency response of under 40 Hz, power-line interference must be eliminated by filtering. Low-pass filters with roll-off above 40 Hz are often used. In some applications, however, the bandpass requirements may extend to one or two kHz, and 50-H_2 or 60-Hz rejection is still required. In such cases a sharply tuned notch filter with a high degree of attenuation is required.

When differential amplifiers are used, a notch filter can be added to each differential line. In this experiment you are presented with the application of a dual-notch filter, each half of which is identical. Figure 28-1 shows the bandpass response and attenuation of the notch filter to be constructed. You will construct, test, and evaluate the attentuation and passband of a (gyrator-type notch filter.

EQUATIONS

$$f_n = \frac{1}{6.28R_2\sqrt{C_1C_2}}$$

where: $R_1 = R_2$; $R_4 = R_5$ (28-1)

$$R_4 = \frac{R_3}{2}$$

Attenuation (dB) $= 20 \log_{10} \dfrac{V_{out}}{V_{in}}$ (28-2)

$$Q = \frac{f_n}{f_h - f_l}$$

where:
f_n = Notch frequency   (28-3)
f_h = High frequency
f_l = Low frequency

MATERIALS REQUIRED

ACTIVE DEVICES:
   1 LM3403
RESISTORS: 5%, 1/4 W
   1 2.7 kΩ
   1 4.7 kΩ
   2 10 kΩ
   1 15 kΩ
   2 10 k potentiometer
CAPACITORS: disc, Mylar, electrolytic, 20%, 25 V
   1 0.1 μF

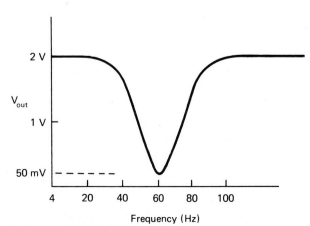

Fig. 28–1. **Attenuation response curve of a notch filter.**

1 1.0 μF
1 2.0 μF
MISCELLANEOUS COMPONENTS:
1 Socket, 14-pin
TEST INSTRUMENTS:

Oscilloscope, dual-trace, 5-in
Function generator, 10 Hz to 1 MHz
Digital multimeter
Power Supply, ± 15 V, 50 mA

TESTS AND MEASUREMENTS

1. Since both circuits are identical, construct only one filter using matched resistors for R_1 and R_2. Potentiometer R_4 is used to tune the circuit to the proper notch frequency and adjust the output waveshape. It can be replaced with a fixed resistor. Potentiometer R_5 requires a 7.5-kΩ resistor (made of two series resistors).

2. Test the notch filter circuit using a 0.1-to-1.0-V p-p sine-wave signal. Determine whether the notch tunes to 60 Hz. Measure input voltage and output voltage and compute the degree of attenuation in decibels.

3. Sketch a frequency-response curve starting with the lowest frequency that your function generator will provide and extend to 1 kHz. Determine the half-voltage point (−6 dB) frequency on each side of the notch and calculate Q.

4. What is the bandwidth of the filter at the (−6-db) point?

5. Most European countries use 50 Hz for power lines. Determine whether the filter notches at 50 Hz, and repeat steps 1 through 4.

6. What is the gain of the filter above and below the notch area?

7. What is the maximum driving signal that can be used without distortion over the frequency range 10 Hz to 1 kHz?

FOR FURTHER RESEARCH

8. With V_{in} = 0.1 V, determine the high-frequency roll-off point (−6 dB).

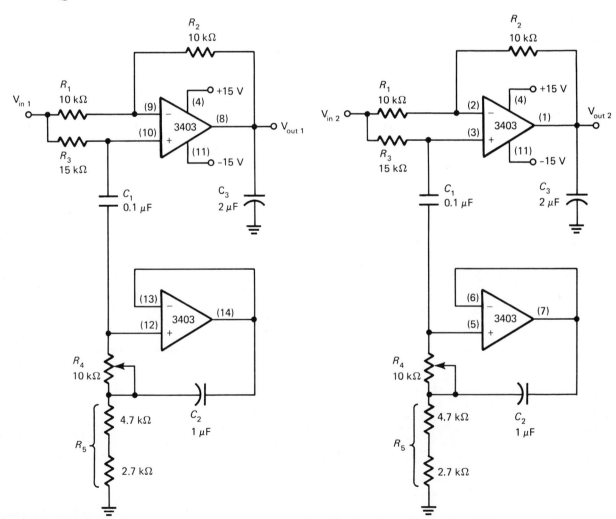

Fig. 28–2. **Dual-notch filters for elimination of 60 Hz in differential amplifiers.**

Test your comprehension of the subject by answering the following questions.

1. The output signal voltage at 100 Hz is 10 mV when the input signal is 3 V. The notch attenuation is minus _____ dB.
2. The center frequency of a notch filter is 100 Hz at 6 dB down, and the frequencies are 95 Hz and 105 Hz. What is the Q?
3. As the Q of the notch increases, the gain of the circuit _____.
4. As capacitor C_1 (Fig. 28-2) is made smaller, the notch frequency goes _____.
5. The gain of the circuit in Fig. 28-2 was found to be _____.

SELF-TEST ANSWERS
1. 49.5 dB
2. 10
3. Increases
4. Higher
5. Unity

29 DIFFERENTIAL AMPLIFIERS

OBJECTIVES

Upon completion of this experiment, unit of study and after the construction of circuitry, testing, and evaluation of data, you will be able to:

1. *Test and evaluate differential amplifiers used in biomedical equipment*

2. *Determine the gain, the frequency response, and the common-mode rejection ratio (CMRR) of such amplifiers*

DISCUSSION

The chip used in this experiment is a CA3051. This device has two identical sections, but only one section is used in this experiment. The differential amplifier used has a double-ended input and output. Either or both outputs can be used. For high-gain applications where a large CMRR is required, two or more such amplifiers can be cascaded. Applications include amplifiers for ECG (or EKG), EEG, and EMG systems.

The differential amplifier is used where a difference voltage has to be amplified in the presence of an interfering common-mode voltage such as 50-Hz or 60-Hz power-line fields, electrical noise, or radiation from other equipment.

When the emitters of two amplifiers are controlled by a constant-current source, which may be in the form of a transistor control, the circuit is described as a *differential amplifier*. Figure 29-1 shows the basic amplifier arrangement. If an out-of-phase voltage is applied to the inputs of amplifiers A and B, the current in A will increase while the current in B will decrease. If both amplifiers and associated parts are identical, the amplifier currents $I_{out\,1}$ and $I_{out\,2}$ will be equal and opposite; hence the net current will be zero and no voltage drop will occur across resistor R_E. Under these conditions the output signal voltage is a function of twice the gain of one amplifier.

If both signals are in phase, such as the pickup from power lines, both $I_{out\,1}$ and $I_{out\,2}$ will increase or decrease simultaneously, thus causing a voltage drop on R_E. This degenerative voltage results in a reduction in amplifier gain.

Of key importance is the ratio of common-mode signal gain (A_{cm}) to differential gain (A_{diff}). This is the CMRR. Expressed as an equation,

$$\text{CMRR} = 20 \log_{10} \frac{A_{cm}}{A_{diff}}$$

(expressed in decibels). Since the ratio A_{cm}/A_{diff} will be less than 1, the computation is made by taking A_{diff}/A_{cm} and expressing the answer in minus decibels. For example, if the ratio is found to be 0.01/10, CMRR is computed as

$$20 \log_{10}\left(\frac{10}{0.01}\right) \quad \text{or} \quad 20 \log_{10}1000 \quad \text{or} \quad 60 \text{ dB}$$

Since it is a loss, the answer is -60 dB. Good amplifiers have CMRRs ranging from 60 to 100 dB. When two or more such amplifiers are cascaded, the CMRR of each can be added. In testing the following circuit, you will (1) measure common-mode rejection (CMR) gain, (2) determine differential gain, (3) determine the CMRR, and (4) determine the frequency response of the amplifier.

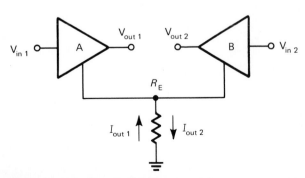

Fig. 29–1. **Principles of differential amplifiers.**

EQUATIONS

$$A = \frac{V_{out}}{V_{in}} \qquad (29\text{-}1)$$

$$CMR = 20 \log_{10} \frac{V_{out}}{V_{in}} \quad (-dB) \qquad (29\text{-}2)$$

$$CMRR = 20 \log_{10} \frac{A_{cm}}{A_{diff}} \quad (dB) \qquad (29\text{-}3)$$

MATERIALS REQUIRED

ACTIVE DEVICES:
   1 CA3051
RESISTORS: 5%, 1/4 W
   1 1 kΩ   **2** 10 kΩ
   1 2.7 kΩ   **2** 100 kΩ

   1 3.3 kΩ
   1 4.7 kΩ
   1 6.8 kΩ
   2 8.2 kΩ
   1 10-kΩ Potentiometer
CAPACITORS: disc, Mylar, electrolytic, 20%, 25 V
   2 0.01 μF
   1 0.05 μF
   1 0.1 μF
   5 100 μF
MISCELLANEOUS COMPONENTS:
   1 Socket 14-pin
TEST INSTRUMENTS:
   Oscilloscope, dual-trace, 5-in
   Function generator, 10 Hz to 1 MHz
   Digital multimeter
   Power supply, ±15 V, 50 mA

TESTS AND MEASUREMENTS

1. Construct the circuit shown in Fig. 29-2 using component values shown. Set V_{CC} to +5 V before connecting it to the circuitry. Set V_{EE} to −5 V.

Single-ended Gain
The following steps provide gain measurements for single-ended input and output:

2. Feed into pin 8 a sine wave of 10 Hz at approximately 10 mV p-p. (If the generator has a DC component, feed the input through a 100-μF capacitor.)

3. Measure the full-gain signal output at pins 6 and 7 and observe the waveshape. What is the output voltage and gain at pin 6 and pin 7? What is the differential gain (pins 6 + 7)?

4. What is the maximum differential gain and maximum single-ended drive signal that the amplifier will accept without overdriving?

5. Try operating the amplifier at ±10 V. What increase in gain takes place with a 10-mV input signal at 10 Hz?

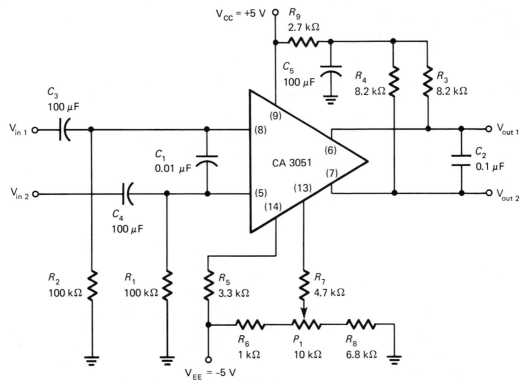

Fig. 29–2. **Differential amplifier with adjustable gain.**

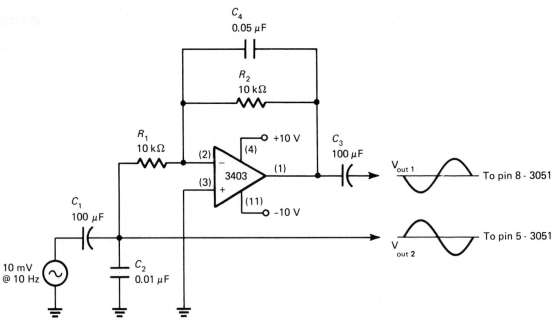

Fig. 29–3. **Phase inverter, unity gain.**

Differential Gain

All measurements are made with P_1 set to provide full gain, $V_{CC} = +10$ V, $V_{EE} = -10$ V.

6. Feed input pins 5 and 8 with a differential signal. This may be obtained by adding the circuit shown in Fig. 29-3 between your generator and the differential amplifier. Adjust the function generator output to 10 mV volts at 10 Hz and feed both inputs ($V_{in\,1}$ and $V_{in\,2}$) of the differential amplifiers (pins 5 and 8). Measure the differential output of your amplifier (if your oscilloscope has a differential input) or measure each output separately and add them together.

By using the chopper setting on the scope, both outputs can be placed one above the other so that the waves just touch. The voltage difference can then be easily determined.

7. What is the differential gain of the amplifier at 10 Hz with a 20-mV differential signal input ($V_{in\,1} = +10$ mV and $V_{in\,2} = -10$ mV)?

Common Mode Rejection

8. Connect the two differential amplifier inputs (pins 8 and 5) together in the manner shown in Fig. 29-4 so that you can determine the common-mode gain. Determine the common-mode amplification A_{cm} by feeding in a signal below the level of saturation at 10 Hz, and determine what input signal is needed to provide the same output as measured in step 5.

9. Compute the common-mode gain (loss).

10. Using common-mode gain and differential gain, compute the CMRR.

Frequency Response

11. Using a 10-mV differential input signal to each amplifier, determine the frequency response of the amplifiers using the 0.01-μF and 0.1-μF capacitors for C_1 and C_2, respectively. Plot your response curve and determine the high-frequency roll-off point at -6 dB.

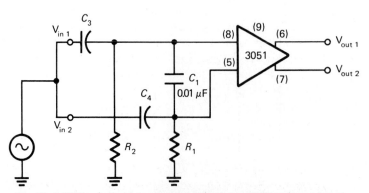

Fig. 29–4. **Method of connecting amplifiers for CMR measurement.**

12. On the same graph paper, plot curves for C_1 removed, for C_2 removed with C_1 installed, and for both C_1 and C_2 removed.

13. What is the -6-dB roll-off on the high end when both capacitors are removed?

14. What components determine the low-frequency roll-off?

NOTE: Do not disassemble the circuitry, as it will be used in Experiment 30.

FOR FURTHER RESEARCH

15. Based on your gain measurements, what gain would you expect if both halves of the CA3051 were connected in cascade to form four amplifiers (two differential pairs)?

16. What would the estimated CMRR be for both amplifiers?

17. What is the purpose of R_9 (2.7 kΩ) and C_5?

18. What is being controlled within the IC by the gain control?

SELF-TEST

Test your comprehension of the subject by answering the following questions.

1. A 1-mV differential input signal produces an output voltage of 0.1 V. If a common-mode input of 2 V produces the same 0.1-V output, what is the CMRR?

2. A differential amplifier, when fed with 2 mV, has a single-ended output of 0.1 V. The differential voltage output is _____.

3. In the circuit shown in Fig. 29-2, R_9–C_5 is a _____.

4. Capacitors C_1 and C_2 in Fig. 29-2 roll-off the _____ frequencies.

5. In a differential amplifier the common mode signal is rejected by _____ in the constant-current emitter circuitry.

SELF-TEST ANSWERS

1. -66 dB.
2. 0.2 V
3. Power-supply bypass
4. High
5. Degeneration

EXPERIMENT 30

ELECTRO-CARDIOGRAM AMPLIFIERS

OBJECTIVES

Upon completion of the study, this experiment, construction of the circuitry, testing, and evaluation of data, you will be able to:

1. *Test and troubleshoot differential amplifiers using integrated circuits in biomedical equipment such as ECG, EEG, EMG, and tachometer recorders*
2. *Design, modify, and adapt high-gain differential amplifier circuits for use in medical equipment*

DISCUSSION

Before proceeding with this experiment, you may wish to re-read Experiment 29 on differential amplifiers. The circuit presented here is an add-on circuit to the previous amplifier. The second half of the CA3051 differential amplifier will be cascaded so that four amplifiers are working in a differential configuration. Since common-mode checks and frequency-response curves were plotted previously, they are not repeated here. Only the overall differential gain and maximum driving signal are determined.

MATERIALS REQUIRED

ACTIVE DEVICES:
    1 CA3051.
RESISTORS: 5%, 1/4 W

1 2.7 kΩ	1 270 kΩ
2 47 kΩ	1 6.8 kΩ
1 3.3 kΩ	4 8.2 kΩ
5 100 kΩ	2 10 kΩ
2 4.7 kΩ	
1 10-kΩ Potentiometer	

CAPACITORS: disc, Mylar, electrolytic, 20%, 25 V
    1 0.01 μF
    2 0.1 μF
    2 0.22 μF
    2 10 μF
    2 25 μF
    1 100 μF

MISCELLANEOUS COMPONENTS:
    1 Socket, 14-pin
TEST INSTRUMENTS:
    Oscilloscope, dual-trace, 5-in
    Function generator, 10 Hz to 1 MHz
    Digital multimeter
    Power supply, $\pm$15 V, 50 mA

TESTS AND MEASUREMENTS

1. Construct the circuit shown in Fig. 30-1 using component values shown and set plus and minus supplies to 10 V. Look at both outputs on your oscilloscope and determine the maximum allowable single-ended input driving signal that can be used at 10 Hz.

NOTE: Most oscilloscopes have a minimum calibration of 10 mV/cm. Either estimate input voltage or design a voltage divider for the input signal. See step 6.

2. Measure the overall differential gain at 10 Hz.

3. Determine the single-ended output voltage and gain using the maximum differential input signal that does not cause saturation or cutoff.

NOTE: Use the unity-gain inverter shown in Experiment 29 for developing the differential input signal; see step 6 for the suggested input voltage divider.

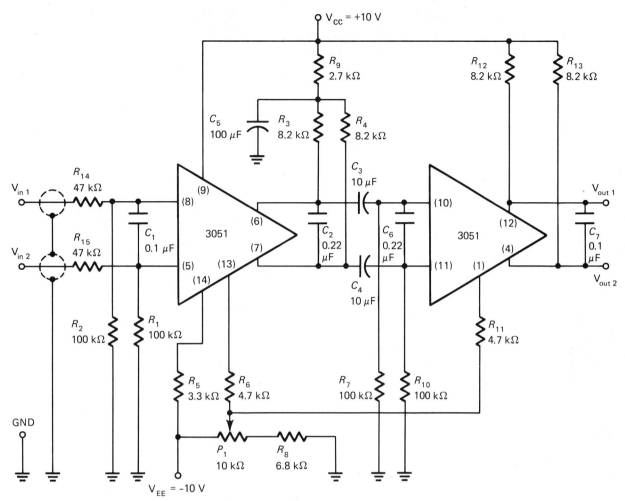

Fig. 30–1. **Cascaded differential amplifiers with variable gain control.**

Measuring ECG

4. Shielded cables are required between inputs 1 and 2 and the subject. The electrodes required should be 3 to 4 cm in diameter and, if possible, silver plated. One possibility would be to use coins. Clean the coins with steel wool or fine sandpaper. Solder each shielded cable (center lead only) to a coin.

Clean an area around the wrist with alcohol and tape a coin in place on each arm. Tape the ground lead to the right ankle (use a coin for contact electrode). The resistance between coin and skin should be under 10,000 Ω. If not, clean the area again and use a little salt water or medical electrode paste.

Make sure *all* equipment is grounded (scope, trainer, leads, voltmeter, etc.) to avoid the possibility of personal injury. When electrodes are in place, set your oscilloscope for 0.1-to-0.5 s/cm sweep and connect one output of your ECG amplifier to your oscilloscope. The vertical amplifiers of your oscilloscope will also increase the gain of your ECG signal.

5. Record the pattern you observe on the scope. If a lot of noise is present, your electrode connections are poorly made. You should observe an ECG pattern similar to the one shown in Fig. 30-2.

As an alternate, you may wish to use the circuit from Experiment 27 for a simulated ECG signal. Use this simulated pulse in place of your own ECG.

FOR FURTHER RESEARCH

6. As most function generators do not have usable output voltages below 1 mV, a voltage divider such as that shown in Fig. 30-3 is suggested. By checking the resistance of 10-kΩ, 10 percent resistors, you will probably have a resistance close to the 9.1-kΩ resistor shown.

7. The circuit shown in Fig. 30-4 can be added to the differential output in order to obtain a single-ended output. Since the MC3403 chip is used for developing a differential input, an unused section of this chip can be used for this circuit. Build and test the circuit.

NOTE: It will be necessary to adjust the gain control to avoid distortion of the output since there is a gain of 27 in this amplifier.

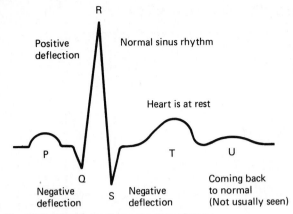

Fig. 30–2. **Electrocardiogram wave-shape.**

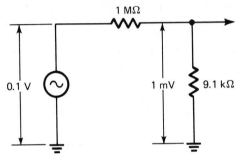

Fig. 30–3. **Voltage-divider circuit.**

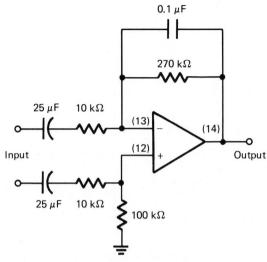

Fig. 30–4. **Differential to single-output amplifier.**

SELF-TEST

Test your comprehension of the subject by answering the following questions. Refer to the circuit shown in Fig. 30-1.

1. The-low frequency response of the circuit is determined by capacitors _____ and _____.

2. The high-frequency response is limited by capacitors _____, _____, _____, and _____.

3. If the CMR of each amplifier section is −40 dB, the total common-mode attenuation is _____.

4. The higher the gain of the amplifiers, the _____ must be the input signal.

5. The differential input resistance of the circuit is no greater than _____.

SELF-TEST ANSWERS
1. C_3 and C_4
2. C_1, C_2, C_6, and C_7
3. −80 dB
4. Smaller
5. 294 kΩ

31 DIFFERENTIAL-INPUT, SINGLE-ENDED-OUTPUT AMPLIFIERS, 60 HZ, FILTERED

OBJECTIVES

Upon completion of this experiment, construction of circuitry, testing, and evaluation of data, you will be able to:

1. *Design, construct, test, and troubleshoot differential amplifiers which make use of operational amplifiers*
2. *Calculate and measure input impedance (resistance) of differential amplifiers which use negative feedback*
3. *Describe the effects of low-input-impedance differential amplifiers*
4. *Determine the effects of coupling capacitors on low-frequency differential amplifiers*
5. *Evaluate the effects of a 60-Hz notch filter*

DISCUSSION

Before proceeding with this experiment, you may wish to review Experiment 29 on differential input instrumentation amplifiers, since the discussion and circuits are applicable to this experiment. This experiment concerns itself primarily with input impedance and associated problems.

The input signal to an amplifier from an ECG is dependent on the amplifier's input impedance and the resistance of the electrodes placed on the patient's body.

$$\text{ECG}_{in} = \frac{\substack{\text{input impedance of} \\ \text{amplifier} \\ \times \text{ ECG voltage}}}{\substack{\text{input impedance of} \\ \text{amplifier} \\ + R \text{ of electrode 1} \\ + R \text{ of electrode 2}}}$$

As can be seen from the equation, amplifier input impedance and electrode resistance greatly affect the output signal from the amplifier.

Suppose, for example, that an amplifier has an input impedance of 100 kΩ, that the electrode's contact to the skin is 50 kΩ (because the electrode paste is of poor quality) instead of being under 10 kΩ, and that the ECG signal is 1 mV. Substituting in the above equation, the signal to the amplifier would be:

$$\begin{aligned} \text{ECG}_{in} &= \frac{R_{in} \text{ of amp} \times \text{ECG volts}}{R_{in} \text{ of amp} + R_{e1} + R_{e2}} \\ &= \frac{1 \times 10^5 \times 1 \times 10^{-3}}{(10 \times 10^4) + (5 \times 10^4) + (5 \times 10^4)} \\ &= \frac{1 \times 10^2}{20 \times 10^4} = 5 \times 10^{-4} = 500 \ \mu\text{V} \end{aligned}$$

This means that only half (50 percent) of the original incoming signal will reach the amplifier. If the contact resistance is reduced to 5kΩ each, 90 percent of the original incoming ECG voltage will reach the amplifier.

The designer of the amplifier cannot be certain that the proper contacts to the skin will be made by the ECG equipment operators. It is important, therefore, that the amplifier's input impedance be made sufficiently high and that the effects of contact resistance are minimized.

The MC3403 used in this experiment has a typical input resistance of 1 MΩ. With two amplifiers configured as a differential pair, the input impedance is 2 MΩ. Consider the effect of poor electrode contact with the skin when this type of amplifier is used:

$$\begin{aligned} \text{ECG}_{in} &= \frac{2 \times 10^6 \times 1 \times 10^{-3}}{(200 \times 10^4) + (5 \times 10^4) + (5 \times 10^4)} \\ &= \frac{2 \times 10^3}{210 \times 10^4} = 9.5 \times 10^{-4} = 950 \ \mu\text{V} \end{aligned}$$

It is clearly seen that only 5 percent of the ECG signal is lost under conditions of poor electrode contact with the skin. Under good conditions of electrode contact with the skin of the patient, less than 1 percent loss can be realized.

In this experiment you will measure the input resistance of the amplifier circuit and determine the phase shift caused by coupling capacitors.

EQUATIONS

$$X_C = \frac{1}{6.28fC} \qquad (31\text{-}1)$$

$$\text{Phase shift } (\Phi) = \text{arc sin } \frac{C}{a} \qquad (31\text{-}2)$$

MATERIALS REQUIRED

ACTIVE DEVICES:
  1 MC3403
  1 TL074

RESISTORS: 5%, 1/4 W
  1 680 Ω
  3 10 kΩ
  2 47 kΩ
  2 100 kΩ
  3 1 MΩ
  1 10-kΩ Potentiometer
CAPACITORS: disc, Mylar, electrolytic, 20%, 25 V
  1 1.02 μF
  2 10 μF
MISCELLANEOUS COMPONENTS:
  1 Socket, 14-pin
TEST INSTRUMENTS:
  Oscilloscope, dual-trace, 5-in
  Function generator, 10 Hz to 1 MHz
  Digital multimeter
  Power supply, ±15V, 50 mA
  Resistance decade box

TESTS AND MEASUREMENTS

In these tests the amplifier's input resistance is determined by placing a variable resistance in series with the input. When the output voltage V_{out} drops to 50 percent, the series resistance R_x is equal to the input resistance of the amplifier.

1. Using the indicated component values, construct the circuit shown in Fig. 31-1. Measure and record static voltages on the used pins of the IC with the inputs V_1 and V_2 grounded.

Set the generator to 10 Hz and apply a signal of 5 to

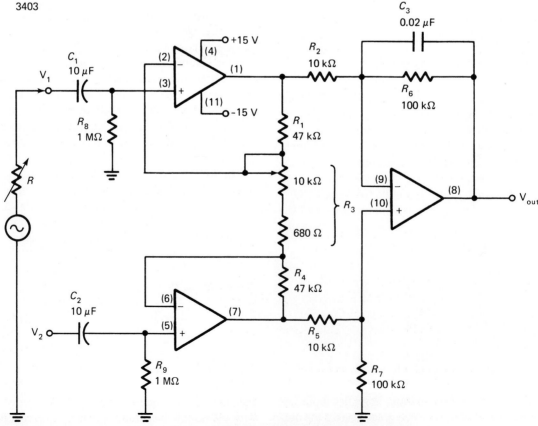

Fig. 31-1. Differential input, single-ended output amplifier.

10 mV to input V_1. Adjust the gain to near maximum and monitor the V_{out}.

2. Insert resistors (a decade box will inject too much 60 Hz noise) in series with the generator and increase resistance values (R_x) until V_{out} is reduced to half its original value. At this point R_x is equal to the input resistance of one-half of the differential amplifier. (A series potentiometer can also be used for finer measurements, but the leads must be kept short.) Measure and record the value of R_x. Determine the value of the total differential input resistance.

3. Ground input V_2 and apply a 2-mV sine wave at 10 Hz to input V_1. Measure V_{out} and calculate the single-ended input gain of the amplifier. Set the gain control at maximum.

NOTE: Since most oscilloscopes have only a 10-mV/cm low scale, the voltage divider circuit shown in Fig. 31-2 will provide the approximate input to V_1.

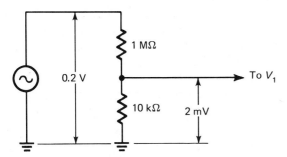

Fig. 31–2. **Voltage-dividing signal.**

Coupling Capacitor Attenuation
A good ECG amplifier should have a minimum frequency response of 0.1 to 50 Hz (established by the American Heart Association). To obtain such a response, the reactance (X_C) value of coupling capacitors in ohms should be 5 percent or less of the input resistance at the lowest frequency.

4. Consider capacitors C_1 and C_2 in Fig. 31-1. Calculate the X_C at 0.1 Hz and determine its percentage of the input resistance.

5. What size of capacitor should be used for C_1 and C_2 to pass frequencies down to 0.1 Hz?

Phase Shift in Coupling Capacitors
Besides attenuation due to the coupling capacitor, phase shift can also occur. This could distort the signal waveshape and give a poor interpretation of the waveshape.

6. Arrange your generator and oscilloscope according to the scheme shown in Fig. 31-3.
NOTE: Some laboratory generators may not go below 10 or 20 Hz; therefore, these tests steps are presented with the results. If your laboratory equipment has the

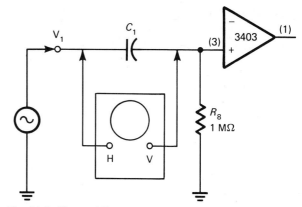

Fig. 31–3. **Phase-shift measurement.**

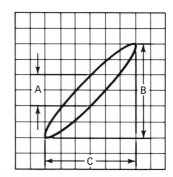

Fig. 31–4. **A coupling circuit with phase shift.**

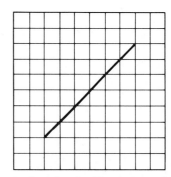

Fig. 31–5. **A coupling circuit without phase shift.**

capabilities required, you are encouraged to conduct the test steps.

7. Substitute a 0.05-μF capacitor for capacitor C_1. Because output voltage is not a concern here, the amplitude of the 10-Hz input signal can be increased as necessary. Observe and sketch the pattern on the oscilloscope. (NOTE: adjust the vertical and horizontal gain and positioning controls so as to center the pattern on the screen). Thus $C_1 = 0.05$ μF (10-Hz input), and phase shift = $\sin \theta = A/B$. Determine the phase shift.

8. The loss due the coupling capacitor is expressed as B (volts)/C (volts). At the lowest frequency the capaci-

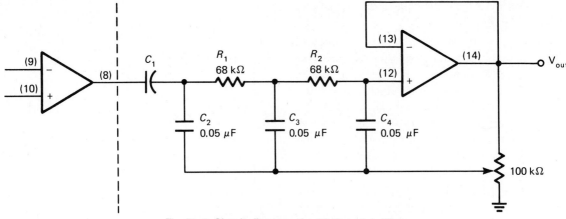

Fig. 31–6. **Circuit diagram of a 60-Hz notch filter.**

tor should produce no loss or phase shift; the desired pattern is a straight line as shown in Fig. 31-5.

FOR FURTHER RESEARCH

9. Construct the 60-Hz filter shown in Fig. 31-6 using the component values indicated. Connect this circuit to the output V_{out} of the circuit shown in Fig. 31-1. Observe the output and describe the effects of the filter on the output voltage using a 10-Hz input at about 2 mV. Test also at 60-Hz.

SELF-TEST

Test your comprehension of the subject by answering the following questions. Refer to Fig. 31-1.

1. The higher the contact resistance for ECG measurements, the _____ the input signal and the higher the _____.

2. The gain of the differential amplifiers is determined by the ratio of resistors _____ to _____.

3. The gain of the output amplifier is computed to be _____.

4. The lower the frequency the more phase shift caused by capacitors _____ and _____.

5. At 0.1 Hz the X_c of C_1 equals _____ Ω.

SELF-TEST ANSWERS
1. Lower, noise
2. R_3 to R_1 ($R_1 = R_4$)
3. 10
4. C_1 and C_2
5. 159.23 k

EXPERIMENT **32** AUDIOMETERS

OBJECTIVES

Upon completion of this experiment, construction of circuitry, testing, and evaluation of data, you will be able to:

1. *Design, test, and evaluate audiometric circuitry using both linear and digital components*

2. *Select and generate the pure audio tones used in audiometry*

3. *Troubleshoot and repair audiometric equipment incorporating linear integrated circuits*

4. *Calibrate, in decibels, attenuators used in audiometers*

DISCUSSION

The human ear responds, remarkably, to a range of frequencies extending from 16 Hz to over 16,000 Hz. Audiometers, however, are standardized to provide test frequencies of 125 Hz, 150 Hz, 500 Hz, 750 Hz, 1000 Hz, 1500 Hz, 2000 Hz, 3000 Hz, 4000 Hz, 6000 Hz, 8000 Hz, and 12,000 Hz. Circuitry in this experiment provides for the generation of tones, the amplification of these discrete tones, and the means to control the intensity of the tone. Referring to Fig. 32-1, tone generation is accomplished using two sections of a 7404 chip, a digital hex inverter, as an astable oscillator. The frequency of oscillation is determined by the value of capacitor C_1 and resistor R_1. One quarter of a quad operational amplifier chip, an MC3403, is resistively coupled to the oscillator to supply the gain of the cir-

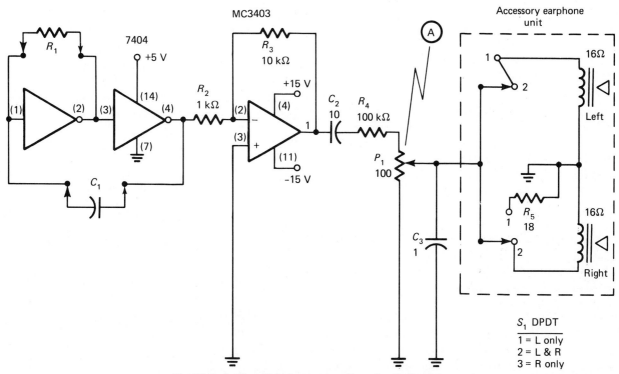

Fig. 32–1. **Audiometric tone-generating circuit diagram.**

cuitry. Additionally, the circuit provides buffering for the oscillator. The output is fed to a voltage-divider attenuator and impedance-matching network for earphones. Attenuation of the tone, within a given range, is determined by the setting of potentiometer P_1. It is noted here that in some cases this function is accomplished through "stepping" of the output intensity as opposed to a variable type of control. Capacitor C_3 filters out high-frequency components and maintains a clear and crisp tone.

EQUATIONS

$$T = RC \qquad (32\text{-}1)$$

$$f_0 \approx \frac{1}{T} \qquad (32\text{-}2)$$

MATERIALS REQUIRED

ACTIVE DEVICES:
1 SN7404
1 MC3403

RESISTORS: 5% 1/4 W
1 18 Ω
1 1 kΩ
1 10 kΩ
1 100 kΩ
Assorted values
1 100-kΩ Potentiometer
CAPACITORS: disc, Mylar, electrolytic, 20%, 25 V
1 1 μF
1 10 μF
Assorted values
MISCELLANEOUS COMPONENTS:
Earphones, 8 to 16 Ω
Speaker, 8 Ω
Switch, DPDT
TEST INSTRUMENTS:
Oscilloscope, dual-trace, 5-in
Function generator, 10 Hz to 1 MHz
Digital multimeter
Power supply, ±15 V, 50 mA

TESTS AND MEASUREMENTS

NOTE: While the circuit to be constructed is shown as termining into a 16-Ω headset, you may use an 8-Ω speaker.

1. Construct the circuit of Fig. 32-1 using component values as indicated. Select the values of C_1 and R_1 to generate a 1-kHz tone. Measure and record static voltages with P_1 set at *minimum*.

2. Substitute other values for C_1 and R_1. Measure and record the period of the generated tones. (**NOTE:** It is necessary in some cases to use two standard-value resistors to obtain the required resistance for R_1.) Explain any difference in the measured and actual periods of the selected tones.

Attenuator Calibration

The audiometer's attenuation control is calibrated in decibels and is referenced to a *zero sensation level*, which represents an *average* of threshold levels of normal ears. Calibration of the attenuator is usually in 5- or 10-dB steps such that 0 dB for each tone generated is the lowest intensity at which the average normal ear can detect the test tone 50 percent of the time. Thus a hearing loss is expressed as the number of decibels in excess of this zero point (up to 100 dB on the dial). A better-than-average normal hearing is provided for on the dial as well (generally −10 db), and a minus sign precedes it.

Since power ratios are independent of sources and load impedances, the expression $10 \log_{10}(P_1/P_2)$ is chosen to determine the number of decibels by which the output levels differ. For example, let the output at test point A (see Fig. 32-1) range 0 to 1 Volt, let the "threshold-level" equal 300 mV across a 10-Ω impedance, and assume that the dial is to calibrate in 10-dB steps.

Then:

1. $P = \dfrac{E^2}{R} = \dfrac{(0.3)^2}{10} = \dfrac{0.09}{10}$

$= 9$ mW $= 0$ dB reference

2. The voltage ratio for a 10-db step $= 3.162$; therefore,

3. $0.3 \times 3.162 = 0.9486$ and

$P = \dfrac{(0.9486)^2}{10} = \dfrac{0.8998}{10} = 89.98$ mW

4. N dB $= 10 \log_{10} \dfrac{P_1}{P_2} = 10 \log_{10} \dfrac{89.98}{9}$

$$= 10 \log_{10} 9.998 = 10 \times 0.9999 = 9.99 \text{ dB}$$

5. Repeat steps 2 through 4 above for the full range of voltage output.

3. Assume the threshold level (0-dB point) to be 5 mW. What is the range of decibels afforded? Provide a chart showing the voltage reading across the earpiece at each decibel setting.

4. Design and provide a drawing of a switching arrangement that enables an audiometrist to select any one of the eight tones generated by the oscillator.

FOR FURTHER RESEARCH

Each of the many sounds ordinarily heard consists of a number of tones, each having a particular pitch and loudness. Detection of the many millions of tones would be a difficult test if the ear were unable to distinguish 1500 different degrees of pitch and 325 different degrees of loudness—one-third of a million different tones.

But when a sound arrives at the ear, it is nothing more than invisible waves of compressed air, the strongest of which are many times fainter than the lightest touch. Just what sort of machine is it that can distinguish one such puff of air from a third of a million others? The simplest form of a hearing machine consists of (1) keys which can be closed by sound waves, (2) wires (nerves) that conduct an electric current to the brain, and (3) the brain. The human hearing mechanism is pictured in Fig. 32-2. It operates in the same manner as the simple one, but instead of one key it has an entire keyboard of 1500 keys. Each key responds to the pressure of tones of *particular frequency* and to no others and produces a sound whose pitch differs from that of any other key on the board. The keys are arranged in such a manner that the end one is closed by tones whose frequency is 16 vibrations per second (the lowest frequency that the human ear can hear) and gives rise to the lowest pitch that humans sense. The next key is closed by tones of a slightly higher frequency and gives rise to a pitch slightly higher than the first. This cycle is repeated on down the line, with the last key at the other end of the board receiving tones of a frequency of 16,000 vibrations per second and giving rise to the shrillest of all sounds. With its 1500 keys this machine can provide such an accurate analysis of the tones contained in the sound waves which strike it that millions of different sounds can be distinguished and correctly identified. A good hearing machine, then, consists of nothing more than a keyboard, wires, and a brain; and the one pictured in Fig. 32-2 would enable a person to hear a great deal. It does, however, lack several refinements, most important of which is protection against damage.

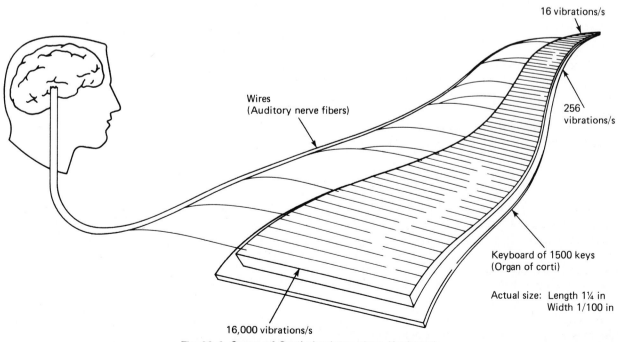

Fig. 32–2. **Organ of Corti simulates piano Keyboard.**

Test your comprehension of the subject by answering the following questions.

1. As R_1 in Fig. 32-1 is made smaller, the frequency of oscillation is _____.
2. Capacitor C_3 in Fig. 32-1 removes _____ frequencies.
3. The signal voltage across an 8-Ω load is 0.3 Volts; this represents a power of _____ W.
4. A power ratio of 1.99 is equal to _____ dB.
5. The typical hearing range for humans is _____ to _____ Hz.

SELF-TEST ANSWERS
1. Higher
2. High
3. 11.25 mW
4. 3 dB
5. 16 to 16,000

EXPERIMENT **33** VOLTAGE-LEVEL COMPARATORS

OBJECTIVES

Upon completion of this experiment, construction of circuitry, testing, and evaluation of data, you will be able to:

1. *Describe the operation of and draw comparator circuits which use linear integrated circuits*
2. *Construct, test, and evaluate comparator-type integrated circuits*
3. *Apply comparator circuits to biomedical systems*

DISCUSSION

In this experiment comparators are applied to the biomedical electronics field. Comparator-type circuits are used where it is desired to determine if an unknown analog voltage equals or exceeds a known reference voltage. The comparator can also be used to convert sine waves and trigger pulses into square waves to serve as a pulse generator.

The comparator makes use of an operational amplifier whose output is fed back to the noninverting input (positive input) in order to provide "snap action" in the output switching. When an operational amplifier is provided with a reference voltage at one input and a trigger or comparing voltage at its other input, the output of the amplifier will rest either at cutoff or saturation. If the amplifier is supplied with +15 V and −15 V, the output will be either plus or minus 15 V, depending on the level of the voltage compared to the reference.

Figure 33-1 shows an inverting voltage comparator. The negative input is supplied with a voltage to be compared with the reference. Since the input is to the negative terminal, the output voltage will be inverted. For the comparator to change its output from high to low, the input voltage must be greater than the reference voltage. There is no upper positive limit as long as the input resistor limits the current to 200 μA or less (depending on the parameters of the operational am-

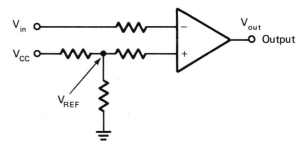

Fig. 33–1. **Inverting-type voltage comparator.**

plifier used). The output of the amplifier can be induced to change quickly (snap action) from one state to the other by providing positive feedback as in Figure 33-3. The input to the amplifier is at the negative terminal, and hence the comparator is of the inverting type. In addition, the feedback network here provides the reference voltage. The reference voltage developed across R_2 is determined as follows:

$$V_{ref} = \frac{R_2}{R_1 + R_2} V_{out}$$

where V_{out} can be either noninverting or inverting. The input signal polarity depends on the resting state of the

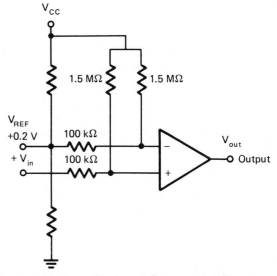

Fig. 33–2. **Non-inverting-type voltage comparator.**

103

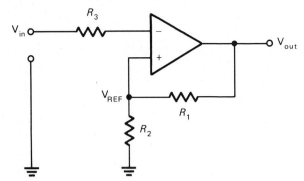

Fig. 33–3. **Voltage comparator with feedback.**

output. If a 10-kΩ resistor is used as feedback from the output, only 1.5 mA will flow when V_{out} is ± 15 V. The value of R_1 can be made equal to 9 kΩ and R_2, to 1 kΩ. The reference voltage would thus have to be plus or minus 1.5 V, depending on the output state, for the switching to occur. The reference level (determined by R_2) can be set as required for comparing voltages up to or near V_{CC}.

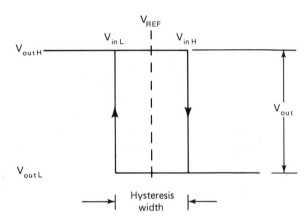

Fig. 33–4. **Hysteresis loop of a comparator.**

The positive-to-negative transition of the output does not follow the same exact path as the negative to positive transition. (This inability to "retrace" exactly on the reverse swing a particular locus of input-output conditions is called *hysteretical behavior.*) The width between the transitions is referred to as the *hysteresis area.* Figure 33-4 shows the dynamic-transfer characteristic curve of the hysteresis area. The smaller the value of the reference voltage (determined by R_2), the smaller is the area width. The equation for the hysteresis area width is:

$$V_{inL} = \frac{R_2}{R_1 + R_2}(V_{out\ H} - V_{ref}) + V_{ref}$$

$$V_{inL} = \frac{R_2}{R_1 + R_2}(V_{out\ L} - V_{ref}) + V_{ref}$$

$$HW = \frac{R_2}{R_1 + R_2}(V_{out\ H} - V_{out\ L})$$

The triggering of the input can be accomplished with a DC or an AC voltage or a sine, a square, or a pulse wave as long as the input voltage exceeds the reference level. Figure 33-5 shows the output (V_{out}) as a result of using a sine-wave trigger. The transfer characteristic loop can be observed on an oscilloscope by using both the vertical and horizontal amplifiers. Figure 33-6 shows how the oscilloscope is to be connected. Since the amplifier input voltage is the smaller, it is connected to the horizontal oscilloscope input. The output of the comparator of Fig. 33-3 can be used as a Schmitt trigger for pulsing circuits that follow. By adjusting the values of R_2, R_1, and R_3 which control the input currents, the input-switching voltage levels, as well as the width of the hysteresis loop, can be established.

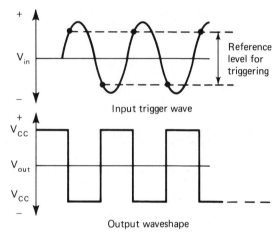

Fig. 33–5. **Triggering level of a comparator.**

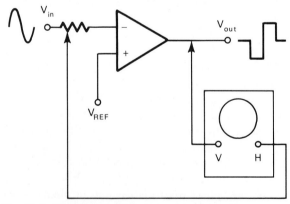

Fig. 33–6. **Oscilloscope connections for viewing hysteresis loop.**

More precise comparators using two or more amplifiers can be arranged. Comparators whose input is a summer can be used to trigger only when the sum of two or more voltages reach the proper trigger level. In the biomedical field the R wave in the ECG *QRST* wave complex is usually higher than the Q, S, or T waves. The peak of the R wave can be used to trigger a comparator so that the remainder of the *QRST* wave complex (Q, S, and T) is eliminated. By using the R peak, a trigger output pulse from the comparator can be derived and used for monitor-tone pulsing, rate counting, alarm delays, and so on. The voltage level of the ECG signal available will determine the reference level of the comparator.

In the experiment that follows, reference levels are established, DC and sine-wave triggering are employed, and the dynamic-transfer curve of hysteresis is investigated.

EQUATIONS

$$V_{ref} = \frac{R_2}{R_1 + R_2} V_{out} \qquad (33\text{-}1)$$

$$HW = \frac{R_2}{R_1 + R_2} (V_{oH} - V_{oL}) \qquad (33\text{-}2)$$

MATERIALS REQUIRED

ACTIVE DEVICES:
1 MC3403

1 2N3904 Transistor
1 1N914 Diode
1 1.7-V Light-emitting diode (LED)
RESISTORS: 5%, 1/4 W
1 47Ω
1 1 kΩ
1 2.7 kΩ
1 10 kΩ
2 33 kΩ
1 100 kΩ
1 10-kΩ Potentiometer
CAPACITORS: disc, Mylar, electrolytic, 20%, 25 V
1 0.002 μF
1 1 μF
MISCELLANEOUS COMPONENTS:
1 Socket, 14-pin
1 Socket, transistor
TEST INSTRUMENTS:
Oscilloscope, dual-trace, 5-in
Function generator, 10 Hz to 1 MHz
Digital multimeter
Power supply, ±15 V, 50 mA

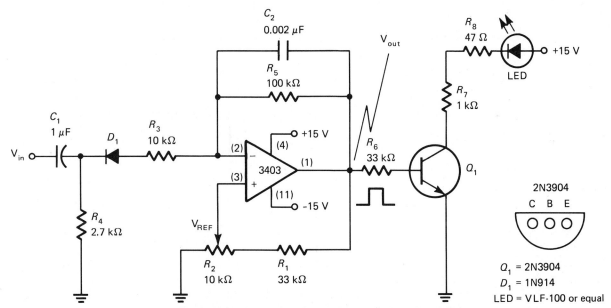

Fig. 33–7. **Evaluation of a comparator and lamp-driving circuit diagram.**

TESTS AND MEASUREMENTS

Static Switching

1. Construct the circuit shown in Fig. 33-7. Set R_2 (reference voltage) to maximum and feed V_{in} with a 10-Hz 2-V square wave, and observe that an output pulse (V_{out}) is produced. Record: (a) input pulse, (b) waveshape across R_4, (c) output pulse amplitude, and (d) output pulse-width range available. Observe effects of pulse width on the LED indicator.

2. Change the input pulse rate to one per second (1 Hz), thus simulating an ECG pulse rate of 60 per minute. Record the waveshape across R_1. What type of circuit is formed by $C_1 R_4$?

3. What is the function of D_1?

4. Assume that V_{in} was the R wave from an ECG signal such as produced by circuits in Experiments 27 through 30. How would you adjust the values of C_1 and/or R_4 so that only the R wave, and not the T wave, produces switching of the comparator?

Sine-wave Triggering

5. Feed a 10-Hz sine wave signal into V_{in}. Determine what voltage level of signal is required to trigger the comparator. Which requires more signal, a square wave or a sine wave? Using a dual-trace oscilloscope, look at the input signal and output simultaneously and compare the patterns to Fig. 33-5. At what peak input voltage level does triggering take place?

6. Leave your generator set at its voltage and decrease or increase the reference voltage until the output drops out. What do you have to do to the input signal in order to retrigger? Change to a triangular wave as a trigger. Overlay one pattern on the other and observe where triggering takes place.

Hysteresis Loop

7. Connect your oscilloscope as shown in Fig. 33-6 and display the hysteresis loop using the 10 Hz sine wave input as the trigger. What is the minimum and maximum width of the loop?

8. Apply a 60-Hz square wave of 1 V p-p to V_{in} (this will simulate an ECG pulse). Monitor the reference voltage at pin 3 and adjust R_2 to obtain a 20-mV reference level. Measure and record the pulse width and amplitude of V_{out}.

9. How could the output pulse obtained in step 8 above be used to drive a relay to control a tone alarm or flashing light monitor?

FOR FURTHER RESEARCH

10. Design a voltage-level comparator which can be used in a patient monitor to indicate the presence of both the ECG signal and blood pressure.

SELF-TEST

Test your comprehension of the subject by answering the following questions.

1. A comparator produces a _____ output whose amplitude is approximately equal to _____.

2. The circuit shown in Fig. 33-7 requires a _____-going pulse.

3. By adjusting R_2, the reference voltage, the level of the _____ wave in a $QRST$ complex can be selected.

4. If the entire $QRST$ passes into a comparator, the output is likely to be a _____ of pulses.

5. The pulse is produced at the output because the amplifier is driven to _____ or _____.

SELF-TEST ANSWERS
1. Pulse, V_{CC}
2. Negative
3. R
4. Series or sequence
5. Cutoff or saturation

EXPERIMENT 34 PULSE KEYERS

OBJECTIVES

Upon completion of this experiment, construction of circuitry, testing, and evaluation of data, you will be able to:

1. *Transfer analog pulse voltages into digital pulses*
2. *Test and troubleshoot pulse circuit amplifiers which use solid-state pulse generators*
3. *Use pulse generators as relay drivers*

DISCUSSION

The circuit to be studied and evaluated is used to change analog voltages such as ECG pulses, pressure pulses, and galvanic skin response (GSR) pulses into rectangular, fast rising, and falling pulses. These rectangular pulses can then be used for rate counting and control functions.

There are many ways in which the circuit can be designed, making use of transistors, linear integrated circuits, or digital integrated circuits. In this experiment pulses from an ECG amplifier or ECG simulator are used to trigger an LM556 timer. The output of the timer is a 10-V pulse which is 0.2 s wide. The output pulse can be used for driving a relay directly, or it can be used in conjunction with other circuitry, such as in experiment 35 for pulse-rate monitoring.

EQUATIONS

$$T = 1.1R_1C_1 \quad \text{(monostable oscillator)} \quad (34\text{-}1)$$

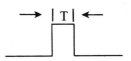

MATERIALS REQUIRED

ACTIVE DEVICES:
  1 LM556.
RESISTORS: 5%, 1/4 W
  2 150 Ω
  1 470 Ω
  1 1 MΩ
CAPACITORS: disc, Mylar, electrolytic, 20%, 25 V
  2 0.01 μF
  1 0.1 μF
  1 500 μF
MISCELLANEOUS COMPONENTS:
  1 Socket, 14-pin
  1 Relay, 3 to 12 V
TEST INSTRUMENTS:
  Oscilloscope, dual-trace, 5-in
  Function generator, 10 Hz to 1 MHz
  Digital multimeter
  Power supply, ±15 V, 50 mA

TESTS AND MEASUREMENTS

NOTE: For the following steps, it is suggested that the ECG simulator (Experiment 27) be used to supply the *negative* trigger pulse to the pulse keyer.

1. Construct the circuit shown in Fig. 34-1 using component values indicated. Measure and record static voltages on used pins of the LM556 chip without a trigger applied at V_{in}.

2. Set the ECG simulator to obtain a trigger pulse of approximately 1 Hz and feed the signal to V_{in} of the pulse keyer. Measure and record the pulse width of V_{out}. Compute the pulse width you would expect at V_{out} for $R_1 = 1$ MΩ and $C_1 = 0.1$ μF.

3. What is the purpose of R_2, C_4, and R_3?

4. Connect a relay to the output of the keyer (pin 5), and determine whether it is keyed at the pulse rate.

NOTE: This circuit is used more extensively in the next experiment (pulse-rate metering); therefore, *do not* disassemble the pulse keyer at this time.

107

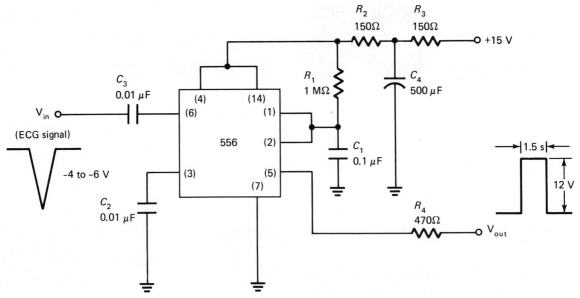

Fig. 34–1. **Pulse keying from an ECG signal.**

SELF-TEST

Test your comprehension of the subject by answering the following questions.

1. The pulse width of the pulse keyer in Fig. 34-1 is determined by _____ and _____.

2. An incoming pulse of _____ volts is needed to trigger the pulse keyer in Fig. 34-1.

3. The *pulse keyer* is another name for a _____ oscillator.

4. The amplitude of the output pulse is determined by the _____.

5. The output pulse period should always be _____ than the period between input pulses.

SELF-TEST ANSWERS
1. R_1 and C_1
2. 3
3. Monostable
4. Power supply
5. Less

35 PULSE-RATE METERING

OBJECTIVES

Upon completion of this experiment, construction of circuitry, testing, and evaluation of data, you will be able to:

1. *Develop and test an integrated circuit amplifier and metering circuit to be used for pulse-rate counting*
2. *Become familiar with pulse filter circuits*
3. *Evaluate how RC filters are used to smooth out pulses*

DISCUSSION

In the biomedical instrumentation field there is a need for pulse-rate averaging and metering. This experiment will provide experiences in working with *RC* filters, integrators, and metering the output of DC amplifiers. The operational amplifier is well suited for this type of application since its input impedance is high and hence will not load down the *RC* filter. The output impedance is low and is well suited for voltmeters, milliameters, and low-resistance recorders. The circuit is designed to handle positive pulses. For negative pulses, the capacitors' polarity would have to be reversed.

In Fig. 35-1 resistors R_1 and R_2 form a voltage divider, and R_2 determines how rapidly the recording output meter returns to 0. Components C_1, C_2, and R_3 form a low-frequency pi filter for producing an average voltage from the incoming pulses. The ratio of R_5 to R_6 determines the gain of the amplifier. For values shown, the gain is approximately 10. With a 1-Hz input signal, the DC voltage at point B is approximately 1.0 V, and output of the amplifier is 10 V. A voltmeter with a 10-to-20-V scale could be calibrated at 6 V for -60 beats per minute (bpm).

Potentiometer P_1 is designed for calibrating the meter and acts as a voltage divider. With no pulse input there will be a DC output voltage of 0 V. Capacitor C_4 provides damping for the meter. The pulse-rate meter is used in ECG recorders and tachometers or in instances where a number of pulses are to be averaged.

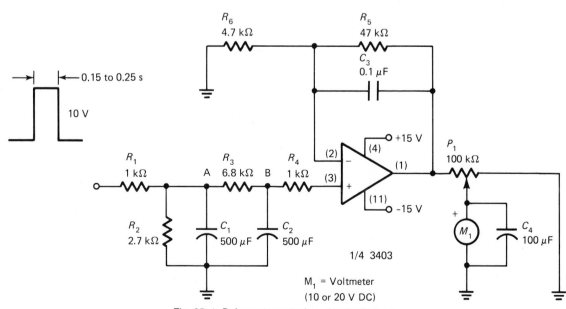

Fig. 35–1. **Pulse-rate metering circuit diagram.**

EQUATIONS

$$T = RC \qquad (35\text{-}1)$$

$$G = \frac{R_f}{R_{in}} = \frac{R_5}{R_6} \qquad (35\text{-}2)$$

$$\text{Beats per minute (bpm)} = \frac{1}{T} \times 60 \qquad (35\text{-}3)$$

MATERIALS REQUIRED

ACTIVE DEVICES:
  1 MC3403
RESISTORS: 5%, 1/4 W
  2 1 kΩ
  1 2.7 kΩ
  1 4.7 kΩ
  1 6.8 kΩ
  1 47 kΩ
  1 100-kΩ Potentiometer
CAPACITORS: disc, Mylar, electrolytic, 20%, 25 V
  1 0.1 μF
  1 100 μF
  2 500 μF
MISCELLANEOUS COMPONENTS:
  1 Socket, 14-pin
  1 Voltmeter, 10 or 20 V DC
TEST INSTRUMENTS:
  Oscilloscope, dual-trace, 5-in
  Function generator, 10 Hz to 1 MHz
  Digital multimeter
  Power supply, ±15 V, 50 mA

TESTS AND MEASUREMENTS

The filter circuit at point A has been designed to pass and filter pulse widths of 0.15 to 0.2 or smaller. Such pulses will produce only minor undulations of the meter vane. A DVM, a VTVM, or a VOM meter can be used for monitoring the pulse rate. If the meter does not have a 10-V range, the calibration control value (P_1) can be adjusted. To test the circuitry, use the pulse output (pin 5) from the pulse keyer (Experiment 34). The input pulse required is +10 V at 0.1 to 0.2 ms.

1. Construct the circuit of Fig. 35-1 using component values as indicated. Measure and record static voltages (without an input pulse). Calibration of the pulse-rate meter should be accomplished at 60 bpm. The ECG simulator (Experiment 27) will produce pulses at the rate of 50 to 75 bpm and hence is used in conjunction with the pulse keyer to conduct further tests in this experiment.

2. Set P_1 of the ECG simulator to obtain a pulse rate of 60 bpm (monitor the pulse-keyer output pulse at pin 5 of the 556 chip). When you are certain that the output of the pulse keyer is precisely 60 bpm, feed this signal to the input of the pulse-rate metering circuit. Adjust the calibration control P_1 for +6 V on the output voltmeter.

3. Adjust P_1 of the ECG simulator to obtain a +5-V-DC reading on the pulse-rate meter. Measure and record the input pulse to the pulse-rate meter. Measure and record the input pulse to the pulse-rate meter at point A and determine the number of beats per minute. *Do not move the calibration control.*

4. Measure and record the voltage at point B. Has the DC level been raised in comparison to the DC level viewed at point A? Use an input pulse rate of 50 bpm.

5. How much gain is provided by the amplifier between point B and the output (pin 1)?

6. With a 60-bpm input signal, disconnect capacitor C_2 and describe the reaction as seen on the output rate meter. Replace C_2 and disconnect capacitor C_1 and describe the meter action.

FOR FURTHER RESEARCH

7. Design a cardiotachometer making use of an ECG input amplifier, pulse keyer or monostable oscillator, and rate meter. If time permits, construct and test your system design.

NOTE: The pulse-rate meter may be disassembled at this time; however, the pulse keyer will be needed for Experiment 36.

SELF-TEST

Test your comprehension of the subject by answering the following questions. Refer to Fig. 35-1.

1. The pulse-rate meter circuit _____ the input voltage pulses.
2. The amplifier's output is a _____-going voltage.
3. The amplifier is connected as a _____.

4. Making R_2 smaller causes the meter to return to 0 _____.

5. By making C_1 and C_2 smaller, the meter will indicate greater _____.

SELF-TEST ANSWERS

1. Averages

2. Positive

3. Noninverter

4. Faster

5. Pulsations

36

ELECTRO-CARDIOGRAM PULSE-BEAT MONITOR, VISUAL INDICATOR

OBJECTIVES

Upon completion of this experiment, construction of circuitry, testing, and evaluation of data, you will be able to:

1. *Test and evaluate circuitry which produces sound and visual indications for patient monitors.*

2. *Use integrated circuit components to produce audio tones*

3. *Use transistors as lamp drivers*

DISCUSSION

Two circuits are studied in this experiment. One circuit generates an audio tone, and the other provides a visual indication of the presence of a pulse. The circuits have application in cardiac monitoring systems where a "beep" or alarm tone and visual indication of pulsing is desired. While linear IC components could have been used, a digital component and transistor provide an alternate circuit design. The intent was to broaden your exposure in the use of other components. All circuits are designed to operate from a positive supply of 5 V.

The lamp driver shown in Fig. 36-1 is quite simple. A transistor is used to drive an LED lamp into the glow condition each time a positive pulse is received at the transistor base. An 8.2-kΩ resistor (R_4) is used to limit base current. At least 2 V of positive pulse is required. This is obtainable from the pulse keyer circuit or pulse delay keyer (Experiments 34 and 37, respectively). The tone generator shown in Fig. 36-1 uses a digital buffer chip (7404 hex inverter) containing six amplifiers. Two amplifiers are used in an astable oscillator circuit which is gated on by the transistor. Three amplifiers of the 7404 are used as drivers for the loudspeaker. The astable oscillator, like the lamp driver, requires a +2-V input pulse.

The astable oscillator frequency is determined by the values of R_3 and C_1, and for values shown, the frequency is approximately 1 kHz. The NPN transistor

(Q_2) gates the circuit on. When no pulse is received at the transistor base, the collector-to-emitter resistance is very high, and the astable circuit will not oscillate. When a pulse is received, the transistor is saturated and the collector-to-emitter resistance drops to a few tenths of an ohm, thus leaving the 150-Ω resistor to determine the frequency of oscillation. The pulse width of the incoming pulse should be at least 0.16. A shorter pulse width will make the tone "chirpy."

Bypass capacitor C_4 removes higher frequencies from the square wave to clear up the tone. Capacitor C_3 keeps DC current out of speaker. Resistors R_1 and R_2 form a voltage divider which limits the incoming drive to the transistor.

MATERIALS REQUIRED

ACTIVE DEVICES:
  1 SN7404
  2 2N3904
  1 1.7-V Light-emitting diode (LED)
RESISTORS: 5%, 1/4 W
  1 47 Ω
  1 150 Ω
  1 8.2 kΩ
  1 10 kΩ
  1 33 kΩ
CAPACITORS: disc, Mylar, electrolytic, 20%, 25 V
  1 0.1 μF
  1 0.22 μF
  1 5 μF
  1 100 μF
MISCELLANEOUS COMPONENTS:
  1 Speaker, 8Ω
  1 Socket, 14-pin
  2 Sockets, transistor
TEST INSTRUMENTS:
  Oscilloscope, dual-trace, 5-in
  Function generator, 10 Hz to 1 MHz
  Digital multimeter
  Power supply, $\pm$15 V, 50 mA

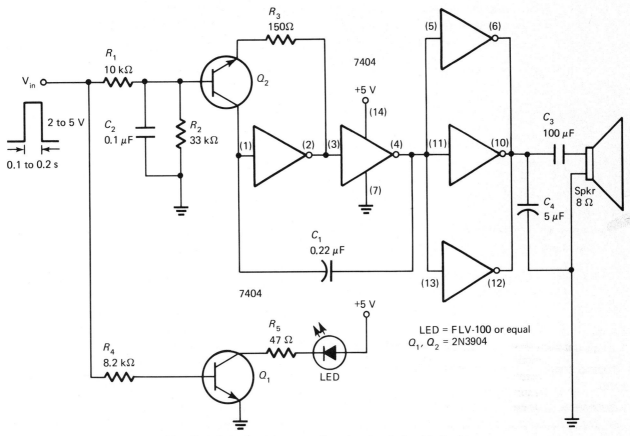

Fig. 36–1. **Pulse-beat tone monitor signal and visual indicator.**

TESTS AND MEASUREMENTS

1. Construct the circuit shown in Fig. 36-1 and arrange for a positive input pulse of 2 to 10 V with a repetition rate of 50 to 100 bpm. The output from pin 5 of the pulse keyer is suggested. Measure and record static voltages.

2. Test the lamp driver circuit first. Does the LED follow the pulse rate? Draw a circuit showing how you would convert this circuit to drive a relay for controlling a higher-voltage lamp.

3. Pulse transistor Q_2 and listen for a tone to be produced. Measure the frequency on your oscilloscope and the waveshape across the speaker. Is the tone chirpy?

4. Try varying the value of R_3. What happens for increased values? What resistance will stop oscillations?

(NOTE: The increase in resistance has the same effect as the collector-to-emitter resistance of Q_2. When Q_2 is turned off, the resistance is high and oscillations cease.)

5. What is the lowest tone frequency you can obtain by varying R_3?

NOTE: This circuitry is to be used in testing Experiment 37. *Do not disassemble it now.* The pulse keyer circuitry can be disassembled at this point, however.

FOR FURTHER RESEARCH

6. How would you add a volume control to the loudspeaker?

7. Design a circuit using linear ICs to provide the same operating functions.

SELF-TEST

Test your comprehension of the subject by answering the following questions. Refer to Fig. 36-1.

1. When Q_1 is driven with a 5-V pulse, the collector voltage of Q_1 is _____ zero.
2. The tone of the oscillator is controlled by the values of _____ and _____.
3. The transistor Q_2 acts as a _____.

4. It is possible to replace Q_1 by one of the other amplifiers on the chip (true or false).

5. The output of the oscillator is a _____ wave.

SELF-TEST ANSWERS

1. Near

2. R_3, and C_1

3. Switch

4. True

5. Square

37

PULSE-DELAY KEYER USING LINEAR/DIGITAL CIRCUITS

OBJECTIVES

Upon completion of this experiment, construction of circuitry, testing, and evaluation of data, you will be able to:

1. *Develop, construct, and test time-delay control circuits which can be used in alarm systems*
2. *Use digital components to make monostable pulsed circuits*
3. *Apply the circuit under study to biomedical instrumentation*

DISCUSSION

The circuits described in this experiment were designed and produced in commercial equipment used for cardiac monitoring. Only part of the system is shown. Basically, the intent is to turn on an alarm tone and automatically stimulate a patient with a pacemaker if the critical cardiac patient has no pulse for a specified period of time (usually 7 to 10 ss). While a cardiac pulse is present a beeping tone and flashing lamp is provided for aural and visual indications. During the immediate crisis of cardiac arrest, the alarm is sounded and the pacemaker applied, or only the alarm is sounded.

Figure 37-1 is a block diagram of how the ECG simulator and the pulse-beat monitor are used with the pulse-delay keyer. The following is a brief description of the operation of the circuit. Referring to Fig. 37-2, capacitor C_2 (100 μF) provides the time delay and is the *key component*. It is charged with a positive voltage applied through resistors R_6 and R_7. The values of C_2, R_6, and R_7 determine the time delay before the alarm action occurs. Resistor R_5 is used to discharge capacitor C_2. While capacitor C_2 is connected to the positive charging source, it is also receiving large negative pulses via the diode which discharges the capacitor. These negative input pulses do not affect the monostable circuit since the monostable circuit needs a positive voltage to actuate it.

If no negative pulses arrive at point A to discharge

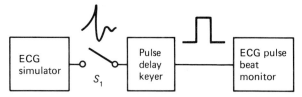

Fig. 37–1. **Block diagram of a pulse-delay keyer.**

capacitor C_2, it will continue to charge in the positive direction. A positive voltage at point B will turn on Q_1, which in turn places a positive voltage pin 2 of the 7400 gate. The result is a production of a positive output pulse for controlling a light, tone, or relay. A relay could be used to control a pacemaker and other emergency equipment and signaling devices. As long as the patient has a cardiac pulse, the voltage on capacitor C_2 rides up and down. Resistors R_6 and R_7 determine how much delay is desired before the alarm is brought on.

MATERIALS REQUIRED

ACTIVE DEVICES:
  1 MC3403
  1 SN7400 or CD 4011
  1 2N5457 FET
  1 1N914 Diode
RESISTORS: 5%, 1/4 W
  1 47 Ω
  2 2.2 kΩ
  1 2.7 kΩ
  1 10 kΩ
  2 47 kΩ
  1 150 kΩ
  1 220 kΩ
  1 1 mΩ
  1 100-kΩ Potentiometer
CAPACITORS: disc, Mylar, electrolytic, 20%, 25 V
  1 50 μF
  1 100 μF
MISCELLANEOUS COMPONENTS:
  2 Sockets, 14-pin
  2 Sockets, transistor

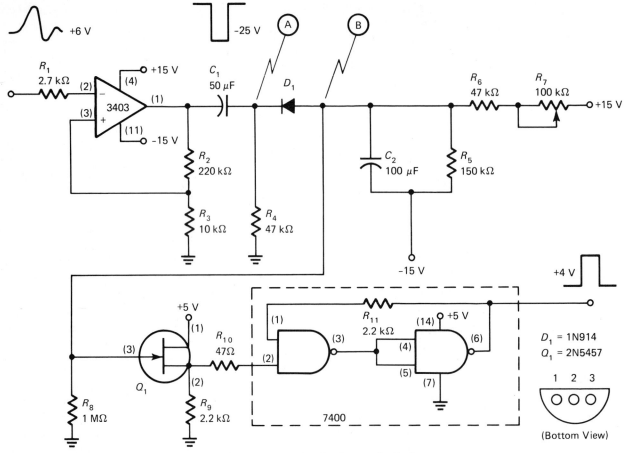

Fig. 37–2. **Comparator and pulse keyer circuit diagram.**

TEST INSTRUMENTS:
Oscilloscope, dual-trace, 5-in
Function generator, 10 Hz to 1 MHz

Digital multimeter
Power supply, ± 15 V, 50 mA

TESTS AND MEASUREMENTS

1. Construct the circuit shown in Fig. 37-2 using component values as indicated. Note that both 15-V and 5-V supplies are being used. Measure and record all static voltages.

2. Using the block diagram and the overall schematic of Fig. 37-3, interconnect the ECG simulator, the circuit of Fig. 37-2, and the ECG pulse-beat monitor. Ensure that the switch is used between the output of the simulator and the input of the pulse-delay keyer.

3. Adjust the amplitude of the ECG simulator to provide the maximum positive input pulse to the pulse delay keyer comparator. Measure and record the output voltage (pin 1) of the comparator.

4. Using a DC coupled oscilloscope, observe the waveshape at point A while pulses are being received. Explain your observations, and measure and record the DC voltage level.

5. Use switch S_1 to disconnect the ECG pulses from the comparator input (this stimulates cardiac arrest)

and record what you observed at point A. Set the delay control R_7 to minimum.

6. Reapply the ECG pulses to the comparator, maintain the delay control at minimum, and observe point B using a DC coupled oscilloscope set to the slowest sweep time. Record your observation of the DC level at point B.

7. Move the delay control R_7 to its maximum insertion resistance and record your observations of the DC level at point B with pulses received.

8. While observing point B, switch off the incoming pulses and record your observations.

9. Measure and record the minimum and maximum delay afforded by control R_7. What is the range of delay provided?

10. How much voltage is required to trigger the monostable circuit? How much output voltage does the monostable provide?

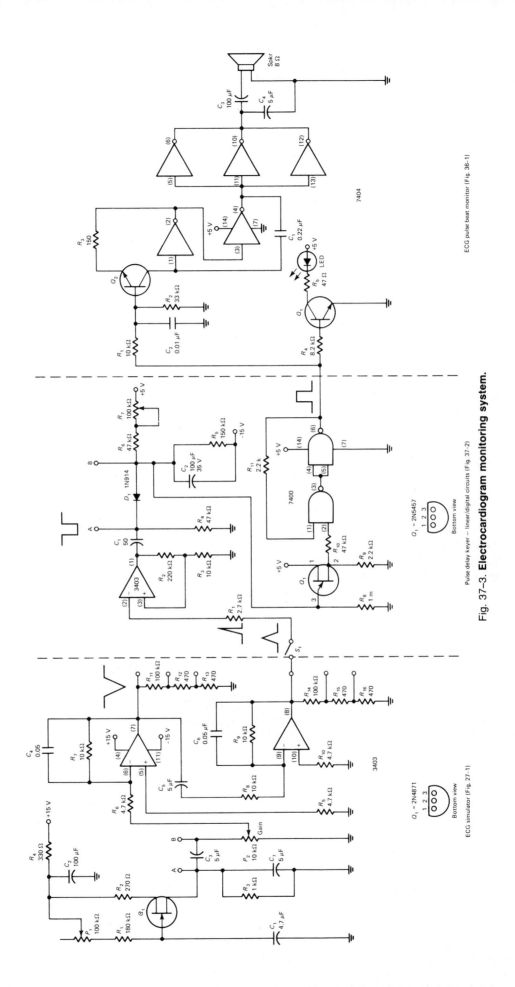

Fig. 37-3. **Electrocardiogram monitoring system.**

117

11. Design a medical monitoring system consisting of differential front-end circuitry, pulse-delay keyer, alarm generator, and visual indicator. Use the same tone generator for beeping (indicating the presence of a heartbeat) as well as for the alarm (indicating the absence of a heartbeat).

SELF-TEST

Test your comprehension of the subject by answering the following questions. Refer to Fig. 37-2.

1. The maximum charge on C_2 could be _____ V.
2. The MC3403 is a _____ circuit.
3. An FET was used for Q_1 since the input to the gate is a _____ resistance which would _____ C_2.
4. The voltage at point B is a series of _____ -going pulses.
5. The time delay is increased by _____ R_7.

SELF-TEST ANSWERS
1. 30
2. Comparator
3. Low, load
4. Positive
5. Increasing

38 PULSE-DELAY KEYER USING LINEAR/TIMER CIRCUITS

OBJECTIVES

Upon completion of this experiment, construction of circuitry, testing, and evaluation of data, you will be able to:

1. *Design and develop circuitry to meet specific requirements*

2. *Test and troubleshoot pulse and timer circuitry used for producing time delay and alarm*

3. *Evaluate pulse alarm-monitoring circuitry*

4. *Apply delayed pulse circuitry to ECG monitoring systems*

DISCUSSION

In Experiment 37 a time-delay circuit combined with a comparator and monostable oscillator was used in a cardiac monitoring system. The circuitry and functions are applicable as well to other types of medical electronic circuitry where time delays or alarms are required. This experiment involves functions similar to those of Experiment 37. However, more modern components are used.

In the experiments thus far you were provided with a circuit description and a schematic of an operable circuit. Emphasis was placed on testing and evaluation. For this experiment, quite a different approach is taken in that you will design the circuitry around predetermined requirements and supply complete details on its ability to meet the specified needs.

Assume that you are a junior engineer assigned to a biomedical electronics equipment designer. You have been given the problem and some ideas, but the circuit design is left to you. It is your responsibility to:

1. Draw the circuit as you think it should be.

2. Make calculations as necessary, using technical data sheets and your previous notes.

3. Build, test, and modify the circuit design as necessary until you get it to perform properly.

4. Thoroughly document the design circuitry and performance tests in an engineering report.

5. Provide details of applications for the circuit you designed.

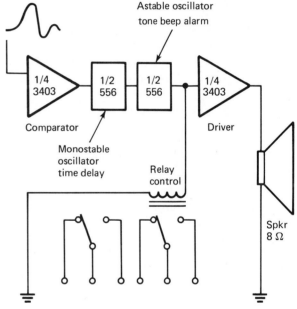

Fig. 38–1. **Block diagram of a pulse-delay relay keyer.**

Circuit Parameters

a. Design a pulse-delay monitor which provides a comparator for ECG voltage-level detection making use of linear-timer components (quad operational amplifier MC3403 and dual timer LM556), and

b. Design the "delay timing" to range from 5 to 10 ss.

c. Provide an audible tone (600 Hz) for a beeper alarm to indicate the presence of an ECG signal.

d. Provide in the design circuitry for automatic activation of a pacemaker and a visual alarm indicator upon cardiac arrest (absence of an ECG signal). A block diagram of the monitor is shown in Fig. 38-1.

NOTES:

1. One or two amplifiers of the MC3403 chip can be used to drive an 8-Ω speaker.

2. The LM556 timer can accommodate both an astable and a monostable oscillator.

MATERIALS REQUIRED

ACTIVE DEVICES:
  1 MC3403
  1 LM556

RESISTORS: 5%, 1/4 W
  Assorted values
CAPACITORS: disc, Mylar, electrolytic, 20%, 25 V
  Assorted values
MISCELLANEOUS COMPONENTS:
  Relay, 6 to 12 V
  2 Sockets, 14-pin
  1 Speaker, 8 Ω
TEST INSTRUMENTS:
  Oscilloscope, dual-trace, 5-in
  Function generator, 10 Hz to 1 MHz
  Digital multimeter
  Power supply, ±15 V, 50 mA

SELF-TEST

Test your comprehension of the subject by answering the following questions.

1. When using an ECG signal for triggering, the _____ pulse is usually used as the trigger.

2. The ECG signal from the body can be taken from across the _____ or from between the _____.

3. An LM556 is a _____ chip.

4. Your own pulse rate is in the range of _____ to _____ bpm (measure it).

5. The time interval between two pulses for 75 bpm is _____.

SELF-TEST ANSWERS
1. *R*
2. Chest, limbs
3. Dual timer
4. 70, 90
5. 0.8 s

EXPERIMENT **39** # PACEMAKER, NERVE STIMULATOR

OBJECTIVES

Upon completion of this experiment, construction of circuitry, testing, and evaluation of data, you will be able to:

1. *Develop circuitry for making a cardiac pacemaker*

2. *Modify circuitry for making a nerve and muscle stimulator*

3. *Test and troubleshoot pacemaker circuits and equipment*

DISCUSSION

There are many ways of designing pacemakers. The circuits shown have been used successfully with pa-

tients both externally and internally. With slight circuit modification, a nerve and muscle stimulator for parotid gland surgery can be provided. The transformer provided for the output of the experimental circuit is suitable for the nerve stimulator but is not large enough to handle the current needed for external pacemaker stimulation.

The circuit consists of a blocking astable oscillator with a variable pulse rate of approximately 50 to 150 beats per minute (bpm) and an output stimulating pulse width of 0.2 to 0.5 ms. The amplitude is variable by a potentiometer and a power transistor drives a step-up transformer for obtaining the voltage for external stimulation. In the commercial pacemaker the power transistor has a capacity of 1 A, and the transformer, of the pulse type, delivers up to 140 V at 0.06 A. A 10-V battery is used for the power source. During the mid

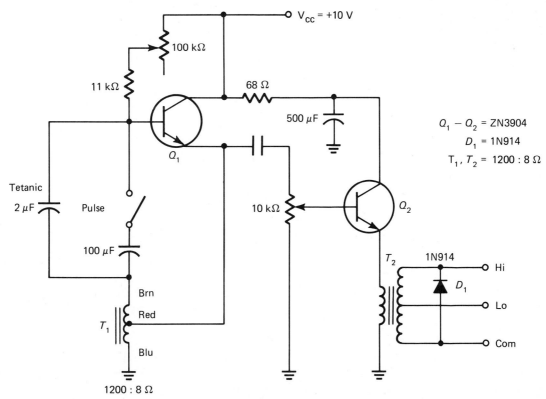

Fig. 39–1. **Blocking oscillator circuit used for nerve stimulation.**

1950s when devices such as the 555 and LM556 were not available, a blocking oscillator circuit was used. This is shown in Fig. 39-1.

The same type of output pulse can be used for the stimulation of nerves and muscles during surgery and for muscle toning. The pulsating wave can be changed to a tetanizing (AC) wave by increasing the frequency to 100 Hz and removing the diode (used for clipping the negative flyback of the transformer). The high-output terminal of the transformer is used for external stimulation, while the low-output terminal is used for exposed tissue during surgery. By placing one electrode (silver or coin disc) which has been moistened on the inner wrist surface and the second on the inner forearm, the high output can be used to locate the nerves that control each finger. If you try this experiment, be sure to start with the amplitude control (P_2) set at 0, and ensure that all equipment is grounded.

In the experiment that follows, a pulsating DC and AC stimulator is tested. The application of the circuit to physiological stimulation is optional.

Design Requirements
The stimulator is to provide:

1. A DC output pulse having a variable rate of approximately 50 to 150 bpm, an amplitude of ≥ 100 V, and a width of 0.2 to 0.5 mV

2. Through switching, change the output stimulating pulses to a form of AC at a rate of 100 Hz

3. Variation in the amplitude of the output stimulating pulse from 0 V to the maximum

EQUATIONS

$$T = t_1 + t_2 = 0.693(R_A + 2R_B)C_1 \qquad (39\text{-}1)$$

$$t_1 = 0.693(R_A + R_B)C_1 \qquad (39\text{-}2)$$

$$t_2 = 0.693R_B C_1 \qquad (39\text{-}3)$$

$$f_0 = \frac{1}{T} = \frac{1.44}{(R_A + 2R_B)C_1} \qquad (39\text{-}4)$$

Beats per minute $= \dfrac{1}{T} \times 60$ where T is in seconds.

$$\qquad (39\text{-}5)$$

MATERIALS AND INSTRUMENTS REQUIRED

ACTIVE DEVICES:
  1 LM556.
  1 2N3638 or 2N3905
  1 1N914 Diode
  1 1.7-V Light-emitting diode (LED)
RESISTORS: 5%, 1/4 W
  Assorted values
CAPACITORS: disc, Mylar, electrolytic, 20%, 25 V
  2 0.01 μF
  1 4.7 μF, tantalytic
  1 50 μF
  1 100 μF
MISCELLANEOUS COMPONENTS:
  1 Socket, 14-pin
  1 Socket, transistor
  1 Switch SPDT
  2 Transformer, 1200 Ω CT/8
TEST INSTRUMENTS:
  Oscilloscope, dual-trace, 5-in
  Function generator, 10 Hz to 1 MHz
  Digital multimeter
  Power supply, $\pm$ 15 V, 50 mA
  Resistance decade box

TESTS AND MEASUREMENTS

1. Let $C_1 = 4.7$ μF and assume that the oscillator should produce a pulse having a 2-ms width. Determine the values of $R_A (P_1 + R_1)$ and R_B to provide the pulse-rate range of 50 to 150 bpm.

2. Determine the values of $R_A (P_1 + R_2)$ and R_B to provide an AC stimulating pulse at the output of 100 Hz.

3. Construct the circuit shown in Fig. 39-2 using standard-value components. Isolate the oscillator and make tests at the output (pin 5) to determine whether the required pulse width and rate range are available. Record the values of components used as well as the measured results.

DC Pulses

4. Measure and record the no-load output pulse voltage and pulse width at 75 bpm (high and low terminals of the transformer) with P_2 set to maximum.

5. Load the high terminal with a 10-kΩ resistor to stimulate the skin contact resistance. What is the maximum voltage and current available for stimulation?

AC Pulses

6. Remove the diode (D_1) and switch the oscillator resistor from R_1 to R_2. The output should be a form of AC. Measure and record the output from the high terminal.

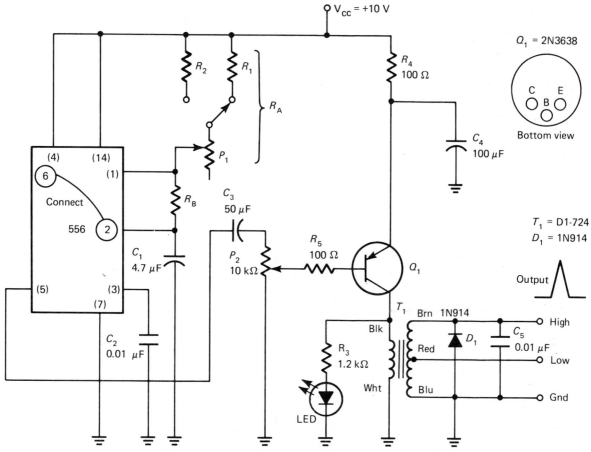

Fig. 39–2. **An AC and DC pulse generator-stimulator.**

7. Ensure that P_1 is set to 0.0 insertion resistance and determine the frequency of the AC stimulating pulses.

8. What is the purpose of diode D_1?

FOR FURTHER RESEARCH

9. The following procedure should be carefully followed:

   a. Set the stimulator to about 100 bpm, DC pulses.
   b. Set P_2 to minimum pulse output.
   c. Connect a lead to an electrode disc (or 5-cent

coin) and secure disc to the underside of your wrist. Use an electrode paste to improve contact.

   d. Secure a second disc with paste about halfway up your forearm.

   e. Slowly increase the amplitude (P_2) until a twitching is observed in one or more fingers.

   f. Vary the pulse rate and also try the AC output. What is the difference in feeling and what effects are noticed?

10. Provide a sketch showing the signals at the base and collector terminals of Q_1 and determine on which slope of the trigger pulse triggering occurs. (**NOTE:** Operate the stimulator in the AC mode.)

SELF-TEST

Test your comprehension of the subject by answering the following questions.

   1. The pulse width is determined by _____.
   2. The value of C_1 is 4.7 μF. Determine R_B when the time between pulses is to be 0.4 s.
   3. Transistor Q_1 is turned on by _____ pulses.
   4. The pulse voltage across the transformer winding (black-white) is 9 V. If the transformer turns ratio is 15:1, the output spike voltage is _____.
   5. Resistor-capacitor R_4C_4 is needed to _____.

SELF-TEST ANSWERS

1. R_1, P_1, and C_1
2. 122.8 kΩ
3. Positive
4. 135 V
5. Reduce pulses to the DC. Power source (V_{CC}).

EXPERIMENT 40 TEMPERATURE AND RESPIRATION

OBJECTIVES

Upon completion of this experiment, construction of circuitry, testing, and evaluation of data, you will be able to:

1. *Develop, construct, and evaluate temperature-measuring circuitry using operational amplifiers*

2. *Utilize astable circuitry and integrators for temperature measurement*

3. *Compare DC and AC circuits for thermistor applications*

DISCUSSION

In Experiment 18, on bridge amplifiers, a thermistor was used in a DC bridge circuit to measure changes in temperature. In this experiment an oscillator is used to feed a thermistor whose resistance changes result in voltage changes which are integrated and fed to a metering circuit. In Experiment 18 a DC voltage provided the source for the bridge, and DC changes resulted in a drift of the metered output. In this experiment an astable (AC) voltage is used to feed the thermistor. The oscillator's output is independent of the supply voltage since the output of the oscillator reaches only 2/3 V_{CC} before recycling; hence the voltage source is somewhat constant.

The thermistor used as the sensor has a negative coefficient; hence as the temperature increases, the resistance of the thermistor decreases. The decrease in resistance is not linear. Each type of thermistor is rated with a coefficient value K, and the resistance of the thermistor follows the equation

$$R = KR_0$$

where R and R_0 are in ohms. The output from the thermistor is a series of pulses whose amplitude in-creases as the resistance decreases. These pulses are averaged by the integrator and appear as a DC output at the meter. The circuit is more stable than the DC bridge and no more complex.

EQUATIONS

$$f_0 = \frac{1}{T} = \frac{1.44}{(R_A + 2R_B)C_1} \qquad (40\text{-}1)$$

$$T = t_1 + t_2 = 0.693(R_A + 2R_B)C_1 \qquad (40\text{-}2)$$

$$D = \frac{R_B}{R_A + 2R_B} \quad \text{where } D \text{ is the duty cycle.} \quad (40\text{-}3)$$

MATERIALS REQUIRED

ACTIVE DEVICES:
   1 LM556.
   1 MC3403
   1 1N914 Diode
RESISTORS: 5%, 1/4 W
   1 680 Ω
   1 4.7 kΩ
   1 6.8 kΩ
CAPACITORS: disc, Mylar, electrolytic, 20%, 25 V
   1 0.001μF
   2 0.01μF
   1 0.1μF
   1 1.0μF
MISCELLANEOUS COMPONENTS:
   2 Sockets, 14-pin.
   1 Thermistor, 100 kΩ
TEST INSTRUMENTS:
   Oscilloscope, dual-trace, 5-in
   Function generator, 10 Hz to 1 MHz
   Digital multimeter
   Power supply, +15 V, 50 mA

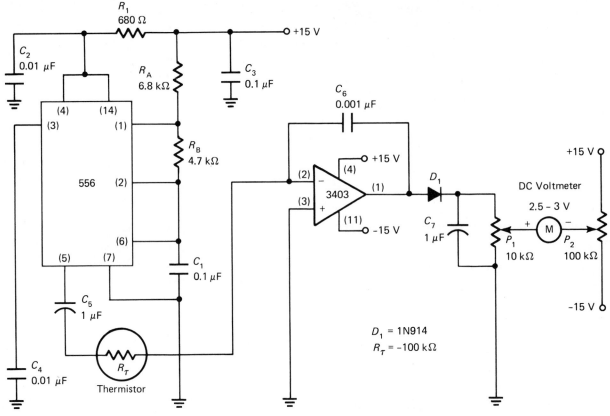

Fig. 40–1. **A circuit diagram for measuring temperature.**

TESTS AND MEASUREMENTS

1. Construct the circuit shown in Fig. 40-1 using component values as indicated. Your laboratory will probably be equipped with a meter that has the required ranges. Measure and record static voltages with P_1 set to minimum and P_2 adjusted to 0 on the meter.

2. After observing the output waveform of the oscillator, provide a sketch that indicates the amplitude and frequency.

3. Using equation (40-3), compute the duty cycle and express the result as a percentage.

4. What type of waveform would you expect to find at pins 1 and 2 of the operational amplifier? Provide a "timing" sketch of your findings.

5. Potentiometer P_1 is used to calibrate the output level of the integrator to full scale when the thermistor is heated. Potentiometer P_2 provides for zero blanching of the meter. Heat the thermistor with your hand and adjust P_1 for full-scale deflection of the meter. Can you obtain full-scale deflection?

(**NOTE:** The meter can be calibrated to any temperature range as desired, depending on the temperature range of the thermistor.

FOR FURTHER RESEARCH

6. Can the circuit be used to measure respiration? If so, how?

7. What is the purpose of components C_2, R_1, and C_3?

SELF-TEST

Test your comprehension of the subject by answering the following questions. Refer to Fig. 40-1.

1. Thermistors are linear, negative-coefficient resistive elements (true-false).
2. The 3403 amplifier integrates the pulses, and its output is an _____ DC voltage.

3. The output to the meter is a _____-going voltage.
4. The bleeder current in the meter-balance potentiometer is _____ mA.
5. The computed frequency of the oscillator is _____ hz.

SELF-TEST ANSWERS
1. False (not linear)
2. Average
3. Positive
4. 0.3
5. 888.8

EXPERIMENT 41 GALVANIC SKIN RESISTANCE (GSR) DETECTOR

OBJECTIVES

Upon completion of this experiment, construction of circuitry, testing, and evaluation of data, you will be able to:

1. *Learn how emotionally induced changes in skin resistance can be measured*
2. *Utilize operational amplifiers to measure physiological changes*
3. *Apply the circuit to optical transducers used for blood flow rate determination*
4. *See how stimulation of the autonomic nervous system (ANS) results in tissue changes whose resistance variation can be measured*
5. *Apply the concepts learned to such applications as lie detectors, degree of alertness, hearing tests, apprehension, fear, panic, and placidity measurements*

DISCUSSION

Human skin resistance varies according to whether the skin is dry, moist, or sweating. These variations can be easily measured since skin resistance ranges from 50 kΩ to 1 MΩ and changes, within 1 percent, as a result of emotional stress. The autonomic nervous system (ANS), which is subject to stimuli from external forces or internal self-stimulating emotional changes, causes reactions, some of which appear as changes in skin resistance. The galvanic skin resistance (GSR) detector or monitor can record such changes in the skin resistance.

Two types of measurement can be made following ANS stimulus: the DC resistance change and the AC resistance change. Depending on the application, either or both measurements are made and used clinically.

The concept of the circuitry is based on measurement of the voltage drop across a resistance through which a constant current is flowing. A high-gain amplifier is used in making the measurement since the voltage changes are in millivolts and microvolts. A current of approximately 10 µA is passed through the resistance of the hand or other skin area, and the voltage drop across the resistance is measured. Since the palm of the hand sweats, electrodes are placed between the palm and the back of the hand in order to measure the change in resistance. In the experiment that follows, only the AC measurement is recorded.

EQUATIONS

$$G = \frac{R_f}{R_{in}} \qquad (41\text{-}1)$$

$$T = RC \qquad (41\text{-}2)$$

MATERIALS REQUIRED

ACTIVE DEVICES:
  1 MC3403
  2 1N914 Diodes
RESISTORS: 5%, 1/4 W

1 1 kΩ	1 470 kΩ
1 2.7 kΩ	1 2.2 MΩ
3 4.7 kΩ	
2 10 kΩ	
1 1.5 kΩ	
1 100 kΩ	
1 10-kΩ Potentiometer	
1 100-kΩ Potentiometer	
1 1-MΩ Potentiometer	

CAPACITORS: disc, Mylar, electrolytic, 20%, 25 V
  1 0.002 µF
  1 0.05 µF
  1 0.1 µF
  1 1 µF
  1 2 µF
  3 100 µF
MISCELLANEOUS COMPONENTS:
  1 Socket, 14-pin
TEST INSTRUMENTS:
  Oscilloscope, dual-trace, 5-in
  Function generator, 10 Hz to 1 MHz
  Digital multimeter
  Power supply, ±15 V, 50 mA

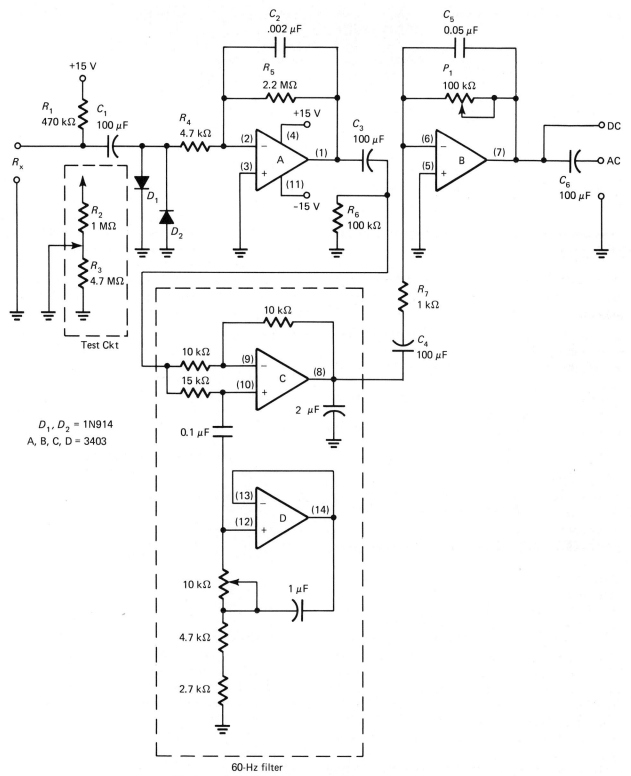

Fig. 41–1. **Galvanic skin response Monitor with 60-Hz filter.**

Referring to Fig. 41-1, resistor R_1 sets the current flow through R_x. For testing, R_2 and R_3 will be used to check the circuit's function; however, the hand will be inserted between the terminals and will become R_x. (CAUTION: Currents of 100 to 200 μA can burn the skin. Make sure your current is in the 5-to-20-μA microampere range.) Measure the skin resistance across your hand. The average is 0.3 to 3 MΩ. Adjust the value of R_1 so that the total current is $R_1 + R_x = 10$ μA.

The change in skin resistance is on the order of 1/10 of 1 percent. Assuming a nominal change in resistance of $1/10 \times 1$ MΩ and 10 μA, the change in voltage due to a stimulus is about 10 mV. If the first amplifier has a gain of 100, the output of the first stage is in the order of 0.1 volt. The output of the second stage, with a gain of 100, is approximately 10 V.

A 60-Hz filter with unity gain at low frequencies is inserted in the circuit between the two amplifiers. The output of amplifier B is observed on a DC coupled oscilloscope. Potentiometer P_1 is a gain control for the second stage. The input pulse is on the order of 0.1 to 0.2 s in width; hence a slow-sweep oscilloscope is required (0.2 to 1.0 s/cm). A voltmeter can also be used to monitor the output.

Gain Measurement

1. Construct the circuit shown in Fig. 41-1. The filter for this circuit is the same as the 60-Hz notch filter constructed in Experiment 28.

2. First measure the overall gain of both amplifiers using a signal of less than 10 mV at frequencies of 5 and 10 Hz. From operational-amplifier gain equations, determine whether the amplifiers are functioning properly. (NOTE: The test circuit components should not be connected at this time.)

AC Galvanic Skin Response

3. Using calibration resistors R_2 and R_3, determine whether the circuit responds to a signal change by momentarily shorting R_3. The output (pin 7) should swing 4 to 6 V.

4. Connect the electrodes with shielded cable to the palm and back of someone's hand, making sure there is adequate pressure so that the electrodes will not move. Measure the skin resistance using an ohmmeter. Moisten the area under the electrodes and again measure the resistance. What resistance value is indicated?

5. Insert cable leads into position R_x. The test circuit resistors, R_2 and R_3, should be removed.

6. Connect a VTVM as well as a DC oscilloscope to the output (pin 7).

7. The person on whom the electrodes are attached should be in a relaxed, seated position with his or her eyes closed. Test the circuit's operation by stimulating the subject. The stimulus can be produced in any number of ways:

  a. Clap your hands behind the subject's head.
  b. Stroke the subject's hair
  c. Rub the leg or the back of the subject's neck.
  d. Use your imagination (depending on the subject) as to how you can excite the subject in order to elicit ANS reaction. The response to look for is a negative swing of the scope's baseline following the stimulus. The output is negative going since the input reflects a drop in resistance due to emotional stress (why not an increase?). The gain control should be set to about midpoint. (If amplifiers are open, the baseline will wander above and below the center when 2 V/cm setting is used.)

8. What is the direction of swing at the output of the first stage?

9. From your measurement of output voltage swing (pin 7) and gain, estimate the percent change in skin resistance.

10. Determine the overall frequency response.

FOR FURTHER RESEARCH

11. The electrodes are formed by using two 5-cent coins (or silver discs) pressure mounted but insulated from each other. A metal spring band can be fabricated, a large insulated chip can be used, or a "C"-shaped clamp can be made to hold the coins firmly in place. Surgical tape or a rubber stamp can also be used. The shielded cable is required because of the high-gain amplifiers and the pickup of stray field currents.

SELF-TEST

Test your comprehension of the subject by answering the following questions.

  1. The human body acts as a volume conductor; hence _____ frequencies will be picked up.
  2. The GSR amplifier has a gain of _____.
  3. The maximum gain of both amplifiers is _____.

4. The two diodes _____ the _____ swings to the amplifiers.

5. If the resistance of the skin tissue inserted into the R_x position is 250,000 Ω, the current through the tissue will be _____.

SELF-TEST ANSWERS
1. 60-Hz
2. 468
3. 46,800
4. Limit the voltage
5. 20.8 μA

1. What are the advantages of using a unijunction transistor as an oscillator rather than using a linear chip?
2. How would you convert single-ended positive pulses to $\pm$ differential pulses?
3. The pulse output of a generator is 1.0 V. The amplifier used requires 100 μV. State the equation you would use for designing an attenuator.
4. What is the typical pulse-rate range in beats per minute (bpm) of an adult?
5. Would a 60-Hz notch filter, which provides 40 dB of attenuation, be considered good or poor?
6. What factors must be considered in the design of a notch filter?
7. If a differential amplifier has an input impedance of 10,000 Ω, what problems may arise if the amplifier is used as an input for ECG monitoring?
8. What bandpass is required by an amplifier to be used for ECG or EEG monitoring?
9. An EEG signal of approximately 10 μV is to be amplified up to 1 V. **a.** How much stage gain is required? **b.** List some chip characteristics to be considered.
10. A quad chip has an intrinsic noise level of 2 μV in each amplifier. If the four amplifiers are arranged in two differential pairs and have a gain of 100, what output noise might you expect?
11. How can you reduce the noise output of a differential amplifier used for ECG measurements?
12. Where is the P wave generated in the heart?
13. What part of the heart generates the QRS complex?
14. What would you consider to be a good hearing range for a young adult (ages 18 to 40 years)?
15. What type of circuit could be used for converting an R wave into a rectangular pulse?
16. What type of pulse must be generated by a pacemaker?
17. What is the resistance range of dry skin?
18. What percentage change in resistance takes place across the hand when a person is subjected to periods of stress?
19. If currents of 1 to 10 mA are passed through the hand while using 1-cm electrodes, what is likely to happen?
20. What is the difference between amplifiers used for ECG, EMG, and EEG monitoring?
21. Provide a pulse-rate block diagram which shows how an ECG signal can be read on a DC meter in the number of beats per minute.
22. List some advantages of using linear quads for differential amplifiers rather than using transistors.
23. A temperature amplifier has a DC output level of 0.6 V. A DC meter is to be connected to the output. Provide a circuit which shows how the DC output can be nulled.
24. What is the frequency range of EEG signals?
25. What should the bandpass range of a GSR amplifier be?

DECIBELS, VOLTAGE, CURRENT, AND POWER RATIOS

APPENDIX A

The decibel, abbreviated dB, is a unit for expressing the ratio of two powers, voltages, or currents. It is used to express the power, voltage, or current gain (or loss).

The basic decibel equation for power is

$$X \text{ dB} = 10 \log \frac{P_{in}}{P_{out}}$$

where P_{out} is power output in watts and P_{in} is power input.

The equation for voltage or current is

$$X \text{ dB} = 20 \log \frac{V_{out}}{V_{in}} \text{ or } \frac{I_{out}}{I_{in}}$$

where V_{out} is output voltage and V_{in} is input voltage.

If the ratio is less than 1, the answer will be in minus ($-$)dB. To express a loss or attenuation, drop the minus sign, and you will have the number of decibels of attenuation. This is the same number of decibels you will get if you invert the ratio.

For example, a gain measurement on a notch filter produced the following data: $V_{in} = 1$ V and $V_{out} = 0.1$ V. What is the degree of attenuation in decibels?

First, invert the ratio. From the voltage ratio 1/0.1 or 10, it is seen in the following table that the decibel value is 20. For this problem the correct answer is 20 dB.

In the table the values listed under the power ratio are the square of those under the voltage ratio.

decibels	voltage and current ratio	power ratio	decibels	voltage and current ratio	power ratio
0.1	1.0116	1.0233	13.0	4.4668	19.953
0.2	1.0233	1.0471	14.0	5.0119	25.119
0.3	1.3351	1.0715	15.0	5.6234	31.623
0.4	1.0471	1.0965	16.0	6.3096	39.811
0.5	1.0593	1.1220	17.0	7.0795	50.119
0.6	1.0715	1.1482	18.0	7.9433	63.096
0.7	1.0839	1.1749	19.0	8.9125	79.433
0.8	1.0965	1.2023	20.0	10.0000	100.00
0.9	1.1092	1.2303	22.0	12.589	158.49
1.0	1.1220	1.2589	24.0	15.849	251.19
1.2	1.1482	1.3183	26.0	19.953	398.11
1.4	1.1749	1.3804	28.0	25.119	630.96
1.6	1.2023	1.4454	30.0	31.623	1000.0
1.8	1.2303	1.5136	32.0	39.811	1584.9
2.0	1.2589	1.5849	34.0	50.119	2511.9
2.2	1.2882	1.6595	36.0	63.096	3981.1
2.4	1.3183	1.7378	38.0	79.433	6309.6
2.6	1.3490	1.8197	40.0	100.000	10^4
2.8	1.3804	1.9055	42.0	125.89	$10^4 \times 1.5849$
3.0	1.4125	1.9953	44.0	158.49	$10^4 \times 2.5119$
3.5	1.4962	2.2387	46.0	199.53	$10^4 \times 3.9811$
4.0	1.5849	2.5119	48.0	251.19	$10^4 \times 6.3096$
4.5	1.6788	2.8184	50.0	316.23	10^5
5.0	1.7783	3.1623	52.0	398.11	$10^5 \times 1.5849$
5.5	1.8836	3.5481	54.0	501.19	$10^5 \times 2.5119$
6.0	1.9953	3.9811	56.0	630.96	$10^5 \times 3.9811$
7.0	2.2387	5.0119	58.0	794.33	$10^5 \times 6.3096$
8.0	2.5119	6.3096	60.0	1,000.00	10^6
9.0	2.8184	7.9433	70.0	3,162.3	10^7
10.0	3.1623	10.0000	80.0	10,000.0	10^8
11.0	3.5481	12.589	90.0	31,623	10^9
12.0	3.9811	15.849	100.0	100,000	10^{10}

2N3638A

KEY

Collector-Emitter Saturation
Voltage at Specified
Collector Current

I_C Units:
A = Amp
M = milliamp

	MATERIAL	POLARITY				MAXIMUM RATINGS						ELECTRICAL CHARACTERISTICS							
TYPE			REPLACE-MENT	REF.	USE	P_D @ 25°C	Ref Point	T_J °C	V_CBO (volts)	V_CE – (volts)	Subscript	h_FE @ I_C (min) (max)		Units	V_CE(SAT) @ I_C (volts)		Units	h_f –	Subscript	f – Units	Subscript

Numerical
Listing
of 2N and 3N
Registered
Type Numbers

S = Silicon
G = Germanium

P = PNP
N = NPN

Type number of redommended
replacement or of nearest
electrical equivalent fully
characterized in this book

Reference device number indicates
specific Data Sheet on
which device is characterized

Common-Emitter DC Short-
Circuit Forward-Current
Transfer Ratio at Specified
Collector Current

I_C Units: A = Amp
M = milliamp
* = microamp
N = nanoamp

Maximum Collector-Emitter Voltage
(Subscript Identifies Condition)

Subscript:
O = V_CEO = Base Open
R = V_CER = Specified Resistance
S = V_CES = Base Shorted
V = V_CEV = Used when only
voltage bias is used
X = V_CEX = Base-Emitter Back
Biased
U = V_CE = Termination Undefined

Small-Signal Forward-Current Transfer Ratio
(E, B or C defines the parameter)

E = h_fe = Common-Emitter Current
Transfer Ratio
B = h_fb = Common-Base Current
Transfer Ratio
C = h_fc = Common-Collector Current
Transfer Ratio

APPLICATION CODE

A = Amplifier
AH = Amplifier, High frequency
AHP = Amplifier, High frequency
power
AL = Amplifier, Light sensitive
AM = Amplifier, Multiple device
AP = Amplifier, Power
S = Switch
SC = Switch, Chopper
SH = Switch, High speed
SHP = Switch, High speed power
SP = Switch, Power

CUTOFF FREQUENCY
Units: K = KHz
M = MHz
G = GHz

(B, E, M or T indicate the Parameter)
B = f_hfb = f_ab = Common-Base Cutoff Frequency
E = f_hfe = f_ae = Common-Emitter Cutoff Frequency
M = f_max = Maximum Frequency of Oscillations
T = f_T = Current Gain - Bandwidth Product

Power Dissipation at 25°C
Units: M = milliwatts
W = Watts
Ref. Point: A, C, J, S, Indicates Ambient,
Case, Junction or Stud

Maximum Collector - Base Voltage

Maximum Operating Junction Temperature

TYPE	MATERIAL	POLARITY	REPLACE-MENT	REF.	USE	P_D @ 25°C	Ref Point	T_J °C	V_CB (volts)	V_CE – (volts)	Subscript	h_FE @ I_C (min)	(max)	Units	V_CE(SAT) @ I_C (volts)		Units	h_f –	Subscript	f – Units	Subscript
2N3638	S	P			SH	0.3W	A	125	25	25	O	30		50M	0.25		50M	25	E	100M	T
2N3638A	S	P			SH	0.3W	A	125	25	25	O	100		50M	0.25		50M	100	E	150M	T
2N3639	S	P	MPS3639	MPS3639	SH	0.2W	A	125	6.0	6.0	O	30	120	10M	0.16		10M			500M	T

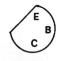
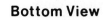

Basing Diagram

Bottom View

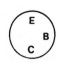

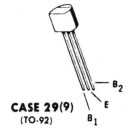

2N4870 (SILICON)
2N4871

CASE 29(9)
(TO-92)

PN unijunction transistors designed for use in pulse and timing circuits, sensing circuits and thyristor trigger circuits.

MAXIMUM RATINGS

RATING	SYMBOL	VALUE	UNIT
RMS Power Dissipation	P_D	300	mW
RMS Emitter Current	I_e	50	mA
Peak-Pulse Emitter Current	i_e	1.5	Amp
Emitter Reverse Voltage	V_{B2E}	30	Volts
Interbase Voltage	V_{B2B1}	35	Volts
Operating Junction Temp. Range	T_J	−65/+125	°C
Storage Temp. Range	T_{stg}	−65/+150	°C

ELECTRICAL CHARACTERISTICS (T_A = 25°C unless otherwise noted)

Characteristic	Fig. No.	Symbol	Min	Typ	Max	Unit
Intrinsic Standoff Ratio* (V_{B2B1} = 10 V) 2N4870 2N4871	4, 7	η^*	0.56 0.70	– –	0.75 0.85	–
Interbase Resistance (V_{B2B1} = 3.0 V, I_E = 0)	10, 11	R_{BB}	4.0	6.0	9.1	k ohms
Interbase Resistance Temperature Coefficient (V_{B2B1} = 3.0 V, I_E = 0, T_A = -65 to +125°C)	11	αR_{BB}	0.10	–	0.90	%/°C
Emitter Saturation Voltage** (V_{B2B1} = 10 V, I_E = 50 mA)		$V_{EB1(sat)}$**	–	2.5	–	Volts
Modulated Interbase Current (V_{B2B1} = 10 V, I_E = 50 mA)		$I_{B2(mod)}$	–	15	–	mA
Emitter Reverse Current (V_{B2E} = 30 V, I_{B1} = 0)	6	I_{EB2O}	–	0.005	1.0	μA
Peak-Point Emitter Current (V_{B2B1} = 25 V)	8, 9	I_P	–	1.0	5.0	μA
Valley-Point Current** (V_{B2B1} = 20 V, R_{B2} = 100 ohms) 2N4870 2N4871	12, 13	I_V**	2.0 4.0	5.0 7.0	– –	mA
Base-One Peak Pulse Voltage 2N4870 2N4871	3, 16	V_{OB1}	3.0 5.0	6.0 8.0	– –	Volts

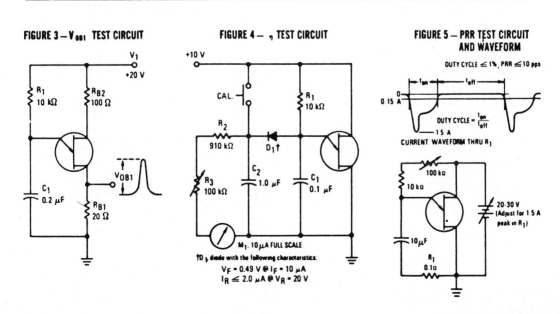

FIGURE 3 — V_{OB1} TEST CIRCUIT

FIGURE 4 — η TEST CIRCUIT

†D_1 diode with the following characteristics:
V_F = 0.49 V @ I_F = 10 μA
I_R ≤ 2.0 μA @ V_R = 20 V

FIGURE 5 — PRR TEST CIRCUIT AND WAVEFORM

DUTY CYCLE ≤ 1%, PRR ≤ 10 pps

DUTY CYCLE = $\frac{t_{on}}{t_{off}}$

CURRENT WAVEFORM THRU R_1

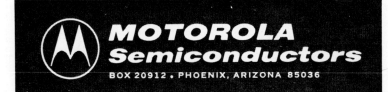

MOTOROLA
Semiconductors

BOX 20912 • PHOENIX, ARIZONA 85036

2N3903
2N3904

NPN SILICON ANNULAR◆ TRANSISTORS

. . . designed for general purpose switching and amplifier applications and for complementary circuitry with types 2N3905 and 2N3906.

- High Voltage Ratings — BV_{CEO} = 40 Volts (Min)
- Current Gain Specified from 100 μA to 100 mA
- Complete Switching and Amplifier Specifications
- Low Capacitance — C_{ob} = 4.0 pF (Max)

NPN SILICON
SWITCHING & AMPLIFIER
TRANSISTORS

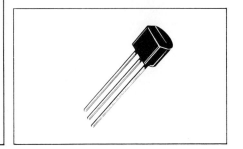

MAXIMUM RATINGS

Rating	Symbol	Value	Unit
*Collector-Base Voltage	V_{CB}	60	Vdc
*Collector-Emitter Voltage	V_{CEO}	40	Vdc
*Emitter-Base Voltage	V_{EB}	6.0	Vdc
*Collector Current	I_C	200	mAdc
Total Power Dissipation @ $T_A = 60^{O}C$	P_D	250	mW
**Total Power Dissipation @ $T_A = 25^{O}C$ Derate above $25^{O}C$	P_D	350 2.8	mW mW/^{O}C
**Total Power Dissipation @ $T_C = 25^{O}C$ Derate above $25^{O}C$	P_D	1.0 8.0	Watts mW/^{O}C
**Junction Operating Temperature	T_J	150	^{O}C
**Storage Temperature Range	T_{stg}	–55 to +150	^{O}C

THERMAL CHARACTERISTICS

Characteristic	Symbol	Max	Unit
Thermal Resistance, Junction to Ambient	$R_{\theta JA}$	357	^{O}C/W
Thermal Resistance, Junction to Case	$R_{\theta JC}$	125	^{O}C/W

*Indicates JEDEC Registered Data

**Motorola guarantees this data in addition to the JEDEC Registered Data.

◆Annular Semiconductors Patented by Motorola Inc.

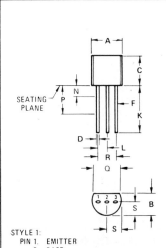

SEATING PLANE

STYLE 1:
PIN 1. EMITTER
 2. BASE
 3. COLLECTOR

DIM	MILLIMETERS		INCHES	
	MIN	MAX	MIN	MAX
A	4.450	5.200	0.175	0.205
B	3.180	4.190	0.125	0.165
C	4.320	5.330	0.170	0.210
D	0.407	0.533	0.016	0.021
F	0.407	0.482	0.016	0.019
K	12.700	–	0.500	–
L	1.150	1.390	0.045	0.055
N	–	1.270	–	0.050
P	6.350	–	0.250	–
Q	3.430	–	0.135	–
R	2.410	2.670	0.095	0.105
S	2.030	2.670	0.080	0.105

CASE 29-02
TO-92

DS 5127 R2

Courtesy of Motorola Inc.

*ELECTRICAL CHARACTERISTICS ($T_A = 25°C$ unless otherwise noted)

Characteristic		Fig. No.	Symbol	Min	Max	Unit
OFF CHARACTERISTICS						
Collector-Base Breakdown Voltage ($I_C = 10~\mu Adc$, $I_E = 0$)			BV_{CBO}	60	-	Vdc
Collector-Emitter Breakdown Voltage (1) ($I_C = 1.0~mAdc$, $I_B = 0$)			BV_{CEO}	40	-	Vdc
Emitter-Base Breakdown Voltage ($I_E = 10~\mu Adc$, $I_C = 0$)			BV_{EBO}	6.0	-	Vdc
Collector Cutoff Current ($V_{CE} = 30~Vdc$, $V_{EB(off)} = 3.0~Vdc$)			I_{CEX}	-	50	nAdc
Base Cutoff Current ($V_{CE} = 30~Vdc$, $V_{EB(off)} = 3.0~Vdc$)			I_{BL}	-	50	nAdc
ON CHARACTERISTICS						
DC Current Gain (1) ($I_C = 0.1~mAdc$, $V_{CE} = 1.0~Vdc$)	2N3903 2N3904	15	h_{FE}	20 40	- -	-
($I_C = 1.0~mAdc$, $V_{CE} = 1.0~Vdc$)	2N3903 2N3904			35 70	- -	
($I_C = 10~mAdc$, $V_{CE} = 1.0~Vdc$)	2N3903 2N3904			50 100	150 300	
($I_C = 50~mAdc$, $V_{CE} = 1.0~Vdc$)	2N3903 2N3904			30 60	- -	
($I_C = 100~mAdc$, $V_{CE} = 1.0~Vdc$)	2N3903 2N3904			15 30	- -	
Collector-Emitter Saturation Voltage (1) ($I_C = 10~mAdc$, $I_B = 1.0~mAdc$)		16, 17	$V_{CE(sat)}$	-	0.2	Vdc
($I_C = 50~mAdc$, $I_B = 5.0~mAdc$)				-	0.3	
Base-Emitter Saturation Voltage (1) ($I_C = 10~mAdc$, $I_B = 1.0~mAdc$)		17	$V_{BE(sat)}$	0.65	0.85	Vdc
($I_C = 50~mAdc$, $I_B = 5.0~mAdc$)				-	0.95	
SMALL-SIGNAL CHARACTERISTICS						
Current-Gain—Bandwidth Product ($I_C = 10~mAdc$, $V_{CE} = 20~Vdc$, $f = 100~MHz$)	2N3903 2N3904		f_T	250 300	- -	MHz
Output Capacitance ($V_{CB} = 5.0~Vdc$, $I_E = 0$, $f = 100~kHz$)		3	C_{ob}	-	4.0	pF
Input Capacitance ($V_{BE} = 0.5~Vdc$, $I_C = 0$, $f = 100~kHz$)		3	C_{ib}	-	8.0	pF
Input Impedance ($I_C = 1.0~mAdc$, $V_{CE} = 10~Vdc$, $f = 1.0~kHz$)	2N3903 2N3904	13	h_{ie}	0.5 1.0	8.0 10	k ohms
Voltage Feedback Ratio ($I_C = 1.0~mAdc$, $V_{CE} = 10~Vdc$, $f = 1.0~kHz$)	2N3903 2N3904	14	h_{re}	0.1 0.5	5.0 8.0	X 10-4
Small-Signal Current Gain ($I_C = 1.0~mAdc$, $V_{CE} = 10~Vdc$, $f = 1.0~kHz$)	2N3903 2N3904	11	h_{fe}	50 100	200 400	-
Output Admittance ($I_C = 1.0~mAdc$, $V_{CE} = 10~Vdc$, $f = 1.0~kHz$)		12	h_{oe}	1.0	40	μmhos
Noise Figure ($I_C = 100~\mu Adc$, $V_{CE} = 5.0~Vdc$, $R_S = 1.0~k~ohms$, $f = 10~Hz$ to $15.7~kHz$)	2N3903 2N3904	9, 10	NF	- -	6.0 5.0	dB
SWITCHING CHARACTERISTICS						
Delay Time ($V_{CC} = 3.0~Vdc$, $V_{BE(off)} = 0.5~Vdc$,		1, 5	t_d	-	35	ns
Rise Time $I_C = 10~mAdc$, $I_{B1} = 1.0~mAdc$)		1, 5, 6	t_r	-	35	ns
Storage Time ($V_{CC} = 3.0~Vdc$, $I_C = 10~mAdc$,	2N3903 2N3904	2, 7	t_s	- -	175 200	ns
Fall Time $I_{B1} = I_{B2} = 1.0~mAdc$)		2, 8	t_f	-	50	ns

(1) Pulse Test: Pulse Width = $300~\mu s$, Duty Cycle = 2.0%.
*Indicates JEDEC Registered Data

FIGURE 1 — DELAY AND RISE TIME EQUIVALENT TEST CIRCUIT

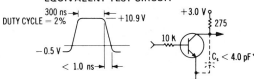

FIGURE 2 — STORAGE AND FALL TIME EQUIVALENT TEST CIRCUIT

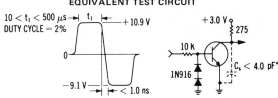

*Total shunt capacitance of test jig and connectors

ⓂMOTOROLA *Semiconductor Products Inc.*

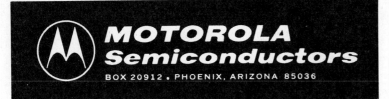

MOTOROLA *Semiconductors*

BOX 20912 • PHOENIX, ARIZONA 85036

2N3905
2N3906

PNP SILICON ANNULAR♦ TRANSISTORS

.... designed for general purpose switching and amplifier applications and for complementary circuitry with types 2N3903 and 2N3904.

- High Voltage Ratings — BV_{CEO} = 40 Volts (Min)
- Current Gain Specified from 100 μA to 100 mA
- Complete Switching and Amplifier Specifications
- Low Capacitance — C_{ob} = 4.5 pF (Max)

PNP SILICON SWITCHING & AMPLIFIER TRANSISTORS

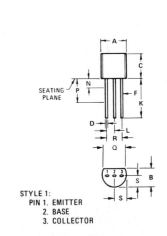

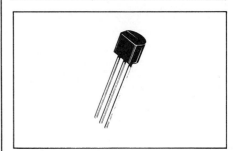

STYLE 1:
PIN 1. EMITTER
    2. BASE
    3. COLLECTOR

DIM	MILLIMETERS		INCHES	
	MIN	MAX	MIN	MAX
A	4.450	5.200	0.175	0.205
B	3.180	4.190	0.125	0.165
C	4.320	5.330	0.170	0.210
D	0.407	0.533	0.016	0.021
F	0.407	0.482	0.016	0.019
K	12.700	–	0.500	–
L	1.150	1.390	0.045	0.055
N	–	1.270	–	0.050
P	6.350	–	0.250	–
Q	3.430	–	0.135	–
R	2.410	2.670	0.095	0.105
S	2.030	2.670	0.080	0.105

CASE 29-02
(TO- 92)

*MAXIMUM RATINGS

Rating	Symbol	Value	Unit
Collector-Base Voltage	V_{CB}	40	Vdc
Collector-Emitter Voltage	V_{CEO}	40	Vdc
Emitter-Base Voltage	V_{EB}	5.0	Vdc
Collector Current	I_C	200	mAdc
Total Power Dissipation @ T_A = 60°C	P_D	250	mW
Total Power Dissipation @ T_A = 25°C Derate above 25°C	P_D	350 2.8	mW mW/°C
Total Power Dissipation @ T_C = 25°C Derate above 25°C	P_D	1.0 8.0	Watt mW/°C
Junction Operating Temperature	T_J	+150	°C
Storage Temperature Range	T_{stg}	−55 to +150	°C

THERMAL CHARACTERISTICS

Characteristic	Symbol	Max	Unit
Thermal Resistance, Junction to Ambient	$R_{\theta JA}$	357	°C/W
Thermal Resistance, Junction to Case	$R_{\theta JC}$	125	°C/W

*Indicates JEDEC Registered Data.
♦Annular semiconductors patented by Motorola Inc.

© MOTOROLA INC., 1973   DS 5128 R2

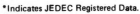

Courtesy of Motorola Inc.

*ELECTRICAL CHARACTERISTICS (T$_A$ = 25°C unless otherwise noted.)

Characteristic		Fig. No.	Symbol	Min	Max	Unit
OFF CHARACTERISTICS						
Collector-Base Breakdown Voltage (I$_C$ = 10 μAdc, I$_E$ = 0)			BV$_{CBO}$	40	—	Vdc
Collector-Emitter Breakdown Voltage (1) (I$_C$ = 1.0 mAdc, I$_B$ = 0)			BV$_{CEO}$	40	—	Vdc
Emitter-Base Breakdown Voltage (I$_E$ = 10 μAdc, I$_C$ = 0)			BV$_{EBO}$	5.0	—	Vdc
Collector Cutoff Current (V$_{CE}$ = 30 Vdc, V$_{BE(off)}$ = 3.0 Vdc)			I$_{CEX}$	—	50	nAdc
Base Cutoff Current (V$_{CE}$ = 30 Vdc, V$_{BE(off)}$ = 3.0 Vdc)			I$_{BL}$	—	50	nAdc
ON CHARACTERISTICS (1)						
DC Current Gain		15	h$_{FE}$			
(I$_C$ = 0.1 mAdc, V$_{CE}$ = 1.0 Vdc)	2N3905			30	—	
	2N3906			60	—	
(I$_C$ = 1.0 mAdc, V$_{CE}$ = 1.0 Vdc)	2N3905			40	—	
	2N3906			80	—	
(I$_C$ = 10 mAdc, V$_{CE}$ = 1.0 Vdc)	2N3905			50	150	
	2N3906			100	300	
(I$_C$ = 50 mAdc, V$_{CE}$ = 1.0 Vdc)	2N3905			30	—	
	2N3906			60	—	
(I$_C$ = 100 mAdc, V$_{CE}$ = 1.0 Vdc)	2N3905			15	—	
	2N3906			30	—	
Collector-Emitter Saturation Voltage		16, 17	V$_{CE(sat)}$			Vdc
(I$_C$ = 10 mAdc, I$_B$ = 1.0 mAdc)				—	0.25	
(I$_C$ = 50 mAdc, I$_B$ = 5.0 mAdc)				—	0.4	
Base-Emitter Saturation Voltage		17	V$_{BE(sat)}$			Vdc
(I$_C$ = 10 mAdc, I$_B$ = 1.0 mAdc)				0.65	0.85	
(I$_C$ = 50 mAdc, I$_B$ = 5.0 mAdc)				—	0.95	
SMALL-SIGNAL CHARACTERISTICS						
Current-Gain — Bandwidth Product			f$_T$			MHz
(I$_C$ = 10 mAdc, V$_{CE}$ = 20 Vdc, f = 100 MHz)	2N3905			200	—	
	2N3906			250	—	
Output Capacitance (V$_{CB}$ = 5.0 Vdc, I$_E$ = 0, f = 100 kHz)		3	C$_{ob}$	—	4.5	pF
Input Capacitance (V$_{BE}$ = 0.5 Vdc, I$_C$ = 0, f = 100 kHz)		3	C$_{ib}$	—	1.0	pF
Input Impedance		13	h$_{ie}$			k ohms
(I$_C$ = 1.0 mAdc, V$_{CE}$ = 10 Vdc, f = 1.0 kHz)	2N3905			0.5	8.0	
	2N3906			2.0	12	
Voltage Feedback Ratio		14	h$_{re}$			X 10^{-4}
(I$_C$ = 1.0 mAdc, V$_{CE}$ = 10 Vdc, f = 1.0 kHz)	2N3905			0.1	5.0	
	2N3906			1.0	10	
Small-Signal Current Gain		11	h$_{fe}$			—
(I$_C$ = 1.0 mAdc, V$_{CE}$ = 10 Vdc, f = 1.0 kHz)	2N3905			50	200	
	2N3906			100	400	
Output Admittance		12	h$_{oe}$			μmhos
(I$_C$ = 1.0 mAdc, V$_{CE}$ = 10 Vdc, f = 1.0 kHz)	2N3905			1.0	40	
	2N3906			3.0	60	
Noise Figure		9, 10	NF			dB
(I$_C$ = 100 μAdc, V$_{CE}$ = 5.0 Vdc, R$_S$ = 1.0 k ohm,	2N3905			—	5.0	
f = 10 Hz to 15.7 kHz)	2N3906			—	4.0	
SWITCHING CHARACTERISTICS						
Delay Time	(V$_{CC}$ = 3.0 Vdc, V$_{BE(off)}$ = 0.5 Vdc	1, 5	t$_d$	—	35	ns
Rise Time	I$_C$ = 10 mAdc, I$_{B1}$ = 1.0 mAdc)	1, 5, 6	t$_r$	—	35	ns
Storage Time	2N3905	2, 7	t$_s$	—	200	ns
(V$_{CC}$ = 3.0 Vdc, I$_C$ = 10 mAdc,	2N3906			—	225	
Fall Time	I$_{B1}$ = I$_{B2}$ = 1.0 mAdc)	2N3905	2, 8	t$_f$	—	60	ns
	2N3906			—	75	

*Indicates JEDEC Registered Data. (1) Pulse Width = 300 μs, Duty Cycle = 2.0 %.

FIGURE 1 – DELAY AND RISE TIME EQUIVALENT TEST CIRCUIT

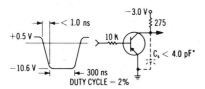

FIGURE 2 – STORAGE AND FALL TIME EQUIVALENT TEST CIRCUIT

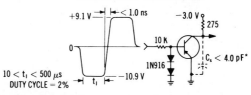

*Total shunt capacitance of test jig and connectors

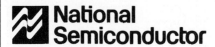 **National Semiconductor**

Operational Amplifiers/Buffers

LM124/LM224/LM324, LM124A/LM224A/LM324A, LM2902
low power quad operational amplifiers

general description

The LM124 series consists of four independent, high gain, internally frequency compensated operational amplifiers which were designed specifically to operate from a single power supply over a wide range of voltages. Operation from split power supplies is also possible and the low power supply current drain is independent of the magnitude of the power supply voltage.

Application areas include transducer amplifiers, dc gain blocks and all the conventional op amp circuits which now can be more easily implemented in single power supply systems. For example, the LM124 series can be directly operated off of the standard +5 V_{DC} power supply voltage which is used in digital systems and will easily provide the required interface electronics without requiring the additional ±15 V_{DC} power supplies.

unique characteristics

- In the linear mode the input common-mode voltage range includes ground and the output voltage can also swing to ground, even though operated from only a single power supply voltage.

- The unity gain cross frequency is temperature compensated.

- The input bias current is also temperature compensated.

advantages

- Eliminates need for dual supplies
- Four internally compensated op amps in a single package
- Allows directly sensing near GND and V_{OUT} also goes to GND
- Compatible with all forms of logic
- Power drain suitable for battery operation

features

- Internally frequency compensated for unity gain
- Large dc voltage gain   100 dB
- Wide bandwidth (unity gain)   1 MHz
  (temperature compensated)
- Wide power supply range:
  Single supply   3 V_{DC} to 30 V_{DC}
  or dual supplies   ±1.5 V_{DC} to ±15 V_{DC}
- Very low supply current drain (800µA) — essentially independent of supply voltage (1 mW/op amp at +5 V_{DC})
- Low input biasing current   45 nA_{DC}
  (temperature compensated)
- Low input offset voltage   2 mV_{DC}
  and offset current   5 nA_{DC}
- Input common-mode voltage range includes ground
- Differential input voltage range equal to the power supply voltage
- Large output voltage   0 V_{DC} to V^+ − 1.5 V_{DC}
  swing

connection diagram

Dual-In-Line and Flat Package

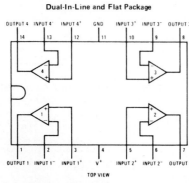

TOP VIEW

Order Number LM124D, LM124AD, LM224D or LM224AD
See NS Package D14E

Order Number LM124F, LM124AF, LM224F or LM224AF
See NS Package F14A

Order Number LM124J, LM124AJ, LM224J, LM224AJ, LM324J, LM324AJ or LM2902J
See NS Package J14A

Order Number LM324N, LM324AN or LM2902N
See NS Package N14A

schematic diagram (Each Amplifier)

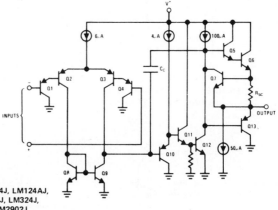

absolute maximum ratings

	LM124/LM224/LM324 LM124A/LM224A/LM324A	LM2902
Supply Voltage, V+	32 VDC or ±16 VDC	26 VDC or ±13 VDC
Differential Input Voltage	32 VDC	26 VDC
Input Voltage	-0.3 VDC to +26 VDC	-0.3 VDC to +26 VDC
Power Dissipation (Note 1)		
Molded DIP	570 mW	570 mW
Cavity DIP	900 mW	
Flat Pack	800 mW	
Output Short-Circuit to GND (One Amplifier) (Note 2) V+ ≤ 15 VDC and TA = 25°C	Continuous	Continuous
Input Current (VIN < -0.3 VDC) (Note 3)	50 mA	50 mA
Operating Temperature Range		-40°C to +85°C
LM324/LM324A	0°C to +70°C	
LM224/LM224A	-25°C to +85°C	
LM124/LM124A	-55°C to +125°C	
Storage Temperature Range	-65°C to +150°C	-65°C to +150°C
Lead Temperature (Soldering, 10 seconds)	300°C	300°C

electrical characteristics ($V^+ = +5.0$ VDC, Note 4)

PARAMETER	CONDITIONS	LM124A MIN	TYP	MAX	LM224A MIN	TYP	MAX	LM324A MIN	TYP	MAX	LM124/LM224 MIN	TYP	MAX	LM324 (LM124A/LM224A/LM324A) MIN	TYP	MAX	LM2902 MIN	TYP	MAX	UNITS
Input Offset Voltage	TA = 25°C, (Note 5)		1	2		1	3		2	3		±2	±5		±2	±7		±2	±7	mVDC
Input Bias Current (Note 6)	IIN(+) or IIN(-), TA = 25°C		20	50		40	80		45	100		45	150		45	250		45	250	nADC
Input Offset Current	IIN(+) - IIN(-), TA = 25°C		2	10		2	15		5	30		±3	±30		±5	±50		±5	±50	nADC
Input Common-Mode Voltage Range (Note 7)	V+ = 30 VDC, TA = 25°C	0		V+-1.5	0		V+-1.5	0		V+-1.5	0		V+-1.5	0		V+-1.5	0		V+-1.5	VDC
Supply Current	RL = ∞, VCC = 30V, (LM2902 VCC = 26V)		1.5	3		1.5	3		1.5	3		1.5	3		1.5	3		1.5	3	mADC
	RL = ∞ On All Op Amps Over Full Temperature Range		0.7	1.2		0.7	1.2		0.7	1.2		0.7	1.2		0.7	1.2		0.7	1.2	mADC
Large Signal Voltage Gain	V+ = 15 VDC (For Large VO Swing) RL ≥ 2 kΩ, TA = 25°C	50	100		50	100		25	100		50	100		25	100			100		V/mV
Output Voltage Swing	RL = 2 kΩ, TA = 25°C (LM2902 RL ≥ 10 kΩ)	0		V+-1.5	0		V+-1.5	0		V+-1.5	0		V+-1.5	0		V+-1.5	0		V+-1.5	VDC
Common Mode Rejection Ratio	DC, TA = 25°C	70	85		70	85		65	85		70	85		65	70		50	70		dB
Power Supply Rejection Ratio	DC, TA = 25°C	65	100		65	100		65	100		65	100		65	100		50	100		dB
Amplifier-to-Amplifier Coupling (Note 8)	f = 1 kHz to 20 kHz, TA = 25°C (Input Referred)		-120			-120			-120			-120			-120			-120		dB
Output Current Source	VIN+ = 1 VDC, VIN- = 0 VDC, V+ = 15 VDC, TA = 25°C	20	40		20	40		20	40		20	40		20	40		20	40		mADC
Output Current Sink	VIN- = 1 VDC, VIN+ = 0 VDC, V+ = 15 VDC, TA = 25°C	10	20		10	20		10	20		10	20		10	20		10	20		mADC
	VIN- = 1 VDC, VIN+ = 0 VDC, TA = 25°C, VO = 200 mVDC	12	50		12	50		12	50		12	50		12	50				•	µADC
Short Circuit to Ground	TA = 25°C, (Note 2)		40	60		40	60		40	60		40	60		40	60		40	60	mADC

electrical characteristics (con't)

PARAMETER	CONDITIONS	LM124A MIN	TYP	MAX	LM224A MIN	TYP	MAX	LM324A MIN	TYP	MAX	LM124/LM224 MIN	TYP	MAX	LM324 MIN	TYP	MAX	LM2902 MIN	TYP	MAX	UNITS
Input Offset Voltage	(Note 5)			4			4			5			±7			±9			±10	mVDC
Input Offset Voltage Drift	$R_S = 0\Omega$		7	20		7	20		7	30		7			7			7		$\mu V/°C$
Input Offset Current	$I_{IN(+)} - I_{IN(-)}$			30			30			75			±100			±150		45	±200	nADC
Input Offset Current Drift			10	200		10	200		10	300		10			10			10		$pADC/°C$
Input Bias Current	$I_{IN(+)}$ or $I_{IN(-)}$		40	100		40	100		40	200		40	300		40	500		40	500	nADC
Input Common-Mode Voltage Range (Note 7)	$V^+ = 30$ VDC	0		V^+-2	0		V^+-2	0		V^+-2	0		V^+-2	0		V^+-2	0		V^+-2	VDC
Large Signal Voltage Gain	$V^+ = +15$ VDC (For Large V_O Swing) $R_L \geq 2$ kΩ	25			25			15			25			15			15			V/mV
Output Voltage Swing V_{OH}	$V^+ = +30$ VDC, $R_L = 2$ kΩ	26			26			26			26			26			22			VDC
	$R_L \geq 10$ kΩ	27	28		27	28		27	28		27	28		27	28		23	24		VDC
V_{OL}	$V^+ = 5$ VDC, $R_L \leq 10$ kΩ		5	20		5	20		5	20		5	20		5	20		5	100	mVDC
Output Current Source	$V_{IN}^+ = +1$ VDC, $V_{IN}^- = 0$ VDC, $V^+ = 15$ VDC	10	20		10	20		10	20		10	20		10	20		10	20		mADC
Sink	$V_{IN}^- = +1$ VDC, $V_{IN}^+ = 0$ VDC, $V^+ = 15$ VDC	10	15		5	8		5	8		5	8		5	8		5	8		mADC
Differential Input Voltage	(Note 7)			V^+			V^+			V^+			V^+			V^+			V^+	VDC

Note 1: For operating at high temperatures, the LM324/LM324A, LM2902 must be derated based on a +125°C maximum junction temperature and a thermal resistance of 175°C/W which applies for the device soldered in a printed circuit board, operating in a still air ambient. The LM224/LM224A and LM124/LM124A can be derated based on a +150°C maximum junction temperature. The dissipation is the total of all four amplifiers—use external resistors, where possible, to allow the amplifier to saturate or to reduce the power which is dissipated in the integrated circuit.

Note 2: Short circuits from the output to V+ can cause excessive heating and eventual destruction. The maximum output current is approximately 40 mA independent of the magnitude of V+. At values of supply voltage in excess of +15 VDC, continuous short-circuits can exceed the power dissipation ratings and cause eventual destruction. Destructive dissipation can result from simultaneous shorts on all amplifiers.

Note 3: This input current will only exist when the voltage at any of the input leads is driven negative. It is due to the collector-base junction of the input PNP transistors becoming forward biased and thereby acting as input diode clamps. In addition to this diode action, there is also lateral NPN parasitic transistor action on the IC chip. This transistor action can cause the output voltages of the op amps to go to the V+ voltage level (or to ground for a large overdrive) for the time duration that an input is driven negative. This is not destructive and normal output states will re-establish when the input voltage, which was negative, again returns to a value greater than −0.3 VDC.

Note 4: These specifications apply for V+ = +5 VDC and −55°C ≤ TA ≤ +125°C, unless otherwise stated. With the LM224/LM224A, all temperature specifications are limited to −25°C ≤ TA ≤ +85°C, the LM324/LM324A temperature specifications are limited to 0°C ≤ TA ≤ +70°C, and the LM2902 specifications are limited to −40°C ≤ TA ≤ +85°C.

Note 5: VO ≅ 1.4 VDC, RS = 0Ω with V+ from 5 VDC to 30 VDC; and over the full input common-mode range (0 VDC to V+ − 1.5 VDC).

Note 6: The direction of the input current is out of the IC due to the PNP input stage. This current is essentially constant, independent of the state of the output so no loading change exists on the input lines.

Note 7: The input common-mode voltage or either input signal voltage should not be allowed to go negative by more than 0.3V. The upper end of the common-mode voltage range is V+ − 1.5V, but either or both inputs can go to +32 VDC without damage (+26 VDC for LM2902).

Note 8: Due to proximity of external components, insure that coupling is not originating via stray capacitance between these external parts. This typically can be detected as this type of capacitive increases at higher frequencies.

typical performance characteristics

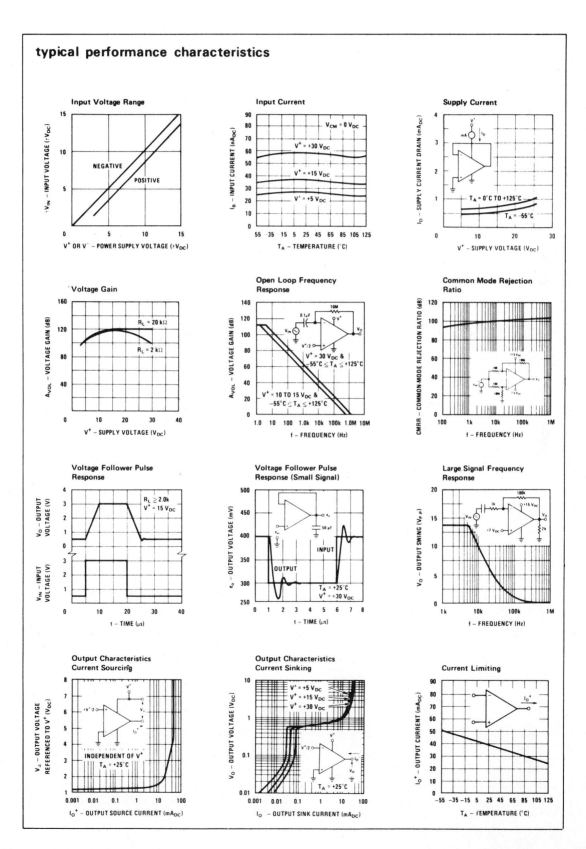

typical performance characteristics (LM2902 only)

Input Current

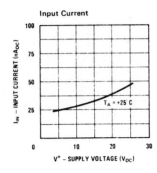

Voltage Gain

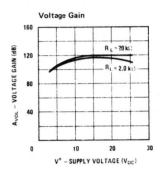

application hints

The LM124 series are op amps which operate with only a single power supply voltage, have true-differential inputs, and remain in the linear mode with an input common-mode voltage of 0 V_{DC}. These amplifiers operate over a wide range of power supply voltage with little change in performance characteristics. At 25°C amplifier operation is possible down to a minimum supply voltage of 2.3 V_{DC}.

The pinouts of the package have been designed to simplify PC board layouts. Inverting inputs are adjacent to outputs for all of the amplifiers and the outputs have also been placed at the corners of the package (pins 1, 7, 8, and 14).

Precautions should be taken to insure that the power supply for the integrated circuit never becomes reversed in polarity or that the unit is not inadvertently installed backwards in a test socket as an unlimited current surge through the resulting forward diode within the IC could cause fusing of the internal conductors and result in a destroyed unit.

Large differential input voltages can be easily accommodated and, as input differential voltage protection diodes are not needed, no large input currents result from large differential input voltages. The differential input voltage may be larger than V^+ without damaging the device. Protection should be provided to prevent the input voltages from going negative more than −0.3 V_{DC} (at 25°C). An input clamp diode with a resistor to the IC input terminal can be used.

To reduce the power supply current drain, the amplifiers have a class A output stage for small signal levels which converts to class B in a large signal mode. This allows the amplifiers to both source and sink large output currents. Therefore both NPN and PNP external current boost transistors can be used to extend the power capability of the basic amplifiers. The output voltage needs to raise approximately 1 diode drop above ground to bias the on-chip vertical PNP transistor for output current sinking applications.

For ac applications, where the load is capacitively coupled to the output of the amplifier, a resistor should be used, from the output of the amplifier to ground to increase the class A bias current and prevent crossover distortion. Where the load is directly coupled, as in dc applications, there is no crossover distortion.

Capacitive loads which are applied directly to the output of the amplifier reduce the loop stability margin. Values of 50 pF can be accommodated using the worst-case non-inverting unity gain connection. Large closed loop gains or resistive isolation should be used if larger load capacitance must be driven by the amplifier.

The bias network of the LM124 establishes a drain current which is independent of the magnitude of the power supply voltage over the range of from 3 V_{DC} to 30 V_{DC}.

Output short circuits either to ground or to the positive power supply should be of short time duration. Units can be destroyed, not as a result of the short circuit current causing metal fusing, but rather due to the large increase in IC chip dissipation which will cause eventual failure due to excessive junction temperatures. Putting direct short-circuits on more than one amplifier at a time will increase the total IC power dissipation to destructive levels, if not properly protected with external dissipation limiting resistors in series with the output leads of the amplifiers. The larger value of output source current which is available at 25°C provides a larger output current capability at elevated temperatures (see typical performance characteristics) than a standard IC op amp.

The circuits presented in the section on typical applications emphasize operation on only a single power supply voltage. If complementary power supplies are available, all of the standard op amp circuits can be used. In general, introducing a pseudo-ground (a bias voltage reference of $V^+/2$) will allow operation above and below this value in single power supply systems. Many application circuits are shown which take advantage of the wide input common-mode voltage range which includes ground. In most cases, input biasing is not required and input voltages which range to ground can easily be accommodated.

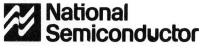

National Semiconductor

Voltage Comparators

LM139/LM239/LM339, LM139A/LM239A/LM339A, LM2901, LM3302 low power low offset voltage quad comparators

general description

The LM139 series consists of four independent precision voltage comparators with an offset voltage specification as low as 2 mV max for all four comparators. These were designed specifically to operate from a single power supply over a wide range of voltages. Operation from split power supplies is also possible and the low power supply current drain is independent of the magnitude of the power supply voltage. These comparators also have a unique characteristic in that the input common-mode voltage range includes ground, even though operated from a single power supply voltage.

Application areas include limit comparators, simple analog to digital converters; pulse, squarewave and time delay generators; wide range VCO; MOS clock timers; multivibrators and high voltage digital logic gates. The LM139 series was designed to directly interface with TTL and CMOS. When operated from both plus and minus power supplies, they will directly interface with MOS logic— where the low power drain of the LM339 is a distinct advantage over standard comparators.

advantages

- High precision comparators
- Reduced V_{OS} drift over temperature

- Eliminates need for dual supplies
- Allows sensing near gnd
- Compatible with all forms of logic
- Power drain suitable for battery operation

features

- Wide single supply voltage range or dual supplies
  LM139 series, 2 V_{DC} to 36 V_{DC} or
  LM139A series, LM2901 ±1 V_{DC} to ±18 V_{DC}
  LM3302 2 V_{DC} to 28 V_{DC}
  or ±1 V_{DC} to ±14 V_{DC}
- Very low supply current drain (0.8 mA) — independent of supply voltage (2 mW/comparator at +5 V_{DC})
- Low input biasing current 25 nA
- Low input offset current ±5 nA
  and offset voltage ±3 mV
- Input common-mode voltage range includes gnd
- Differential input voltage range equal to the power supply voltage
- Low output 250 mV at 4 mA saturation voltage
- Output voltage compatible with TTL, DTL, ECL, MOS and CMOS logic systems

schematic and connection diagrams

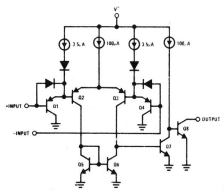

Dual-In-Line and Flat Package

TOP VIEW

Order Number LM139D, LM139AD, LM239D or LM239AD
See NS Package D14E

Order Number LM139J, LM139AJ, LM239J, LM239AJ, LM339J, LM339AJ, LM2901J or LM3302J
See NS Package J14A

Order Number LM139F, LM139AF, LM239F or LM239AF
See NS Package F14A

Order Number LM339N, LM339AN, LM2901N or LM3302N
See NS Package N14A

typical applications (V⁺ = 5.0 V_{DC})

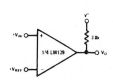

Basic Comparator

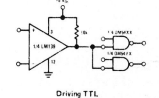

Driving CMOS

Driving TTL

absolute maximum ratings

	LM139/LM239/LM339 LM139A/LM239A/LM339A LM2901	LM3302
Supply Voltage, V^+	36 V_{DC} or ±18 V_{DC}	28 V_{DC} or ±14 V_{DC}
Differential Input Voltage	36 V_{DC}	28 V_{DC}
Input Voltage	−0.3 V_{DC} to +36 V_{DC}	−0.3 V_{DC} to +28 V_{DC}
Power Dissipation (Note 1)		
Molded DIP	570 mW	570 mW
Cavity DIP	900 mW	
Flat Pack	800 mW	
Output Short-Circuit to GND, (Note 2)	Continuous	Continuous
Input Current ($V_{IN} < −0.3$ V_{DC}), (Note 3)	50 mA	50 mA
Operating Temperature Range		
LM339A	0°C to +70°C	−40°C to +85°C
LM239A	−25°C to +85°C	
LM2901	−40°C to +85°C	
LM139A	−55°C to +125°C	
Storage Temperature Range	−65°C to +150°C	−65°C to +150°C
Lead Temperature (Soldering, 10 seconds)	300°C	300°C

electrical characteristics ($V^+ = 5$ V_{DC}, Note 4)

PARAMETER	CONDITIONS	LM139A MIN	TYP	MAX	LM239A, LM339A MIN	TYP	MAX	LM139 MIN	TYP	MAX	LM239, LM339 MIN	TYP	MAX	LM2901 MIN	TYP	MAX	LM3302 MIN	TYP	MAX	UNITS
Input Offset Voltage	$T_A = 25°C$, (Note 9)		±1.0	±2.0		±1.0	±2.0		±2.0	±5.0		±2.0	±5.0		±2.0	±7.0		±3	±20	mV_{DC}
Input Bias Current	$I_{IN(+)}$ or $I_{IN(-)}$ with Output in Linear Range, $T_A = 25°C$, (Note 5)		25	100		25	250		25	100		25	250		25	250		25	500	nA_{DC}
Input Offset Current	$I_{IN(+)} - I_{IN(-)}$, $T_A = 25°C$		±3.0	±25		±5.0	±50		±3.0	±25		±5.0	±50		±5	±50		±3	±100	nA_{DC}
Input Common-Mode Voltage Range	$T_A = 25°C$, (Note 6)	0		V^+-1.5	0		V^+-1.5	0		V^+-1.5	0		V^+-1.5	0		V^+-1.5	0		V^+-1.5	V_{DC}
Supply Current	$R_L = \infty$ on all Comparators, $T_A = 25°C$		0.8	2.0		0.8	2.0		0.8	2.0		0.8	2.0		0.8	2.0		0.8	2	mA_{DC}
	$R_L = \infty$, $V^+ = 30V$, $T_A = 25°C$														1	2.5				mA_{DC}
Voltage Gain	$R_L \geq 15$ kΩ, $V^+ = 15$ V_{DC} (To Support Large V_O Swing), $T_A = 25°C$	50	200		50	200			200			200		25	100		2	30		V/mV
Large Signal Response Time	$V_{IN} = $ TTL Logic Swing, $V_{REF} = 1.4$ V_{DC}, $V_{RL} = 5$ V_{DC}, $R_L = 5.1$ kΩ, $T_A = 25°C$		300			300			300			300			300			300		ns
Response Time	$V_{RL} = 5$ V_{DC}, $R_L = 5.1$ kΩ, $T_A = 25°C$, (Note 7)		1.3			1.3			1.3			1.3			1.3			1.3		µs
Output Sink Current	$V_{IN(-)} \geq 1$ V_{DC}, $V_{IN(+)} = 0$, $V_O \leq 1.5$ V_{DC}, $T_A = 25°C$	6.0	16		6.0	16		6.0	16		6.0	16		6.0	16		6.0	16		mA_{DC}
Saturation Voltage	$V_{IN(-)} \geq 1$ V_{DC}, $V_{IN(+)} = 0$, $I_{SINK} \leq 4$ mA, $T_A = 25°C$		250	400		250	400		250	400		250	400			400		250	500	mV_{DC}
Output Leakage Current	$V_{IN(+)} \geq 1$ V_{DC}, $V_{IN(-)} = 0$, $V_O = 5$ V_{DC}, $T_A = 25°C$		0.1			0.1			0.1			0.1			0.1			0.1		nA_{DC}

electrical characteristics (con't)

PARAMETER	CONDITIONS	LM139A			LM239A, LM339A			LM139			LM239, LM339			LM2901			LM3302			UNITS
		MIN	TYP	MAX	MIN	TYP	MAX	MIN	TYP	MAX	MIN	TYP	MAX	MIN	TYP	MAX	MIN	TYP	MAX	
Input Offset Voltage	(Note 9)			4.0			4.0			9.0			9.0		9	15		9	40	mV_{DC}
Input Offset Current	$I_{IN}(+) - I_{IN}(-)$			±100			±150			±100			±150		50	200			300	nA_{DC}
Input Bias Current	$I_{IN}(+)$ or $I_{IN}(-)$ with Output in Linear Range			300			400			300			400		200	500			1000	nA_{DC}
Input Common-Mode Voltage Range		0		V^+-2.0	0		V^+-2.0	0		V^+-2.0	0		V^+-2.0	0		V^+-2.0	0		V^+-2.0	V_{DC}
Saturation Voltage	$V_{IN}(-) \geq 1\ V_{DC}$, $V_{IN}(+) = 0$, $I_{SINK} \leq 4$ mA			700			700			700			700		400	700			700	mV_{DC}
Output Leakage Current	$V_{IN}(+) \geq 1\ V_{DC}$, $V_{IN}(-) = 0$, $V_O = 30\ V_{DC}$			1.0			1.0			1.0			1.0			1.0			1.0	μA_{DC}
Differential Input Voltage	Keep all V_{IN}'s $\geq 0\ V_{DC}$ (or V^- if used). (Note 8)			V^+			V^+			36			36			V^+			V_{CC}	V_{DC}

Note 1: For operating at high temperatures, the LM339/LM339A, LM2901, LM3302 must be derated based on a 125°C maximum junction temperature and a thermal resistance of 175°C/W which applies for the device soldered in a printed circuit board, operating in a still air ambient. The LM239 and LM139 must be derated based on a 150°C maximum junction temperature. The low bias dissipation and the "ON-OFF" characteristic of the outputs keeps the chip dissipation very small ($P_D \leq 100$ mW), provided the output transistors are allowed to saturate.

Note 2: Short circuits from the output to V^+ can cause excessive heating and eventual destruction. The maximum output current is approximately 20 mA independent of the magnitude of V^+.

Note 3: This input current will only exist when the voltage at any of the input leads is driven negative. It is due to the collector-base junction of the input PNP transistors becoming forward biased and thereby acting as input diode clamps. In addition to this diode action, there is also lateral NPN parasitic transistor action on the IC chip. This transistor action can cause the output voltages of the comparators to go to the V^+ voltage level (or to ground for a large overdrive) for the time duration that an input is driven negative. This is not destructive and normal output states will re-establish when the input voltage, which was negative, again returns to a value greater than −0.3 V_{DC}.

Note 4: These specifications apply for V^+ = 5 V_{DC} and $-55°C \leq T_A \leq +125°C$, unless otherwise stated. With the LM239/LM239A, all temperature specifications are limited to $-25°C \leq T_A \leq +85°C$, the LM339/LM339A temperature specifications are limited to $0°C \leq T_A \leq +70°C$, and the LM2901, LM3302 temperature range is $-40°C \leq T_A \leq +85°C$.

Note 5: The direction of the input current is out of the IC due to the PNP input stage. This current is essentially constant, independent of the state of the output so no loading change exists on the reference or input lines.

Note 6: The input common-mode voltage or either input signal voltage should not be allowed to go negative by more than 0.3V. The upper end of the common-mode voltage range is V^+ −1.5V, but either or both inputs can go to +30 V_{DC} without damage.

Note 7: The response time specified is for a 100 mV input step with 5 mV overdrive. For larger overdrive signals 300 ns can be obtained, see typical performance characteristics section.

Note 8: Positive excursions of input voltage may exceed the power supply level. As long as the other voltage remains within the common-mode range, the comparator will provide a proper output state. The low input voltage state must not be less than −0.3 V_{DC} (or 0.3 V_{DC} below the magnitude of the negative power supply, if used).

Note 9: At output switch point, $V_O \cong 1.4\ V_{DC}$. $R_S = 0\Omega$ with V^+ from 5 V_{DC}; and over the full input common-mode range (0 V_{DC} to V^+ −1.5 V_{DC}).

Note 10: For input signals that exceed V_{CC}, only the overdriven comparator is affected. With a 5V supply, V_{IN} should be limited to 25V max, and a limiting resistor should be used on all inputs that might exceed the positive supply.

typical performance characteristics LM139/LM239/LM339, LM139A/LM239A/LM339A, LM3302

typical performance characteristics LM2901

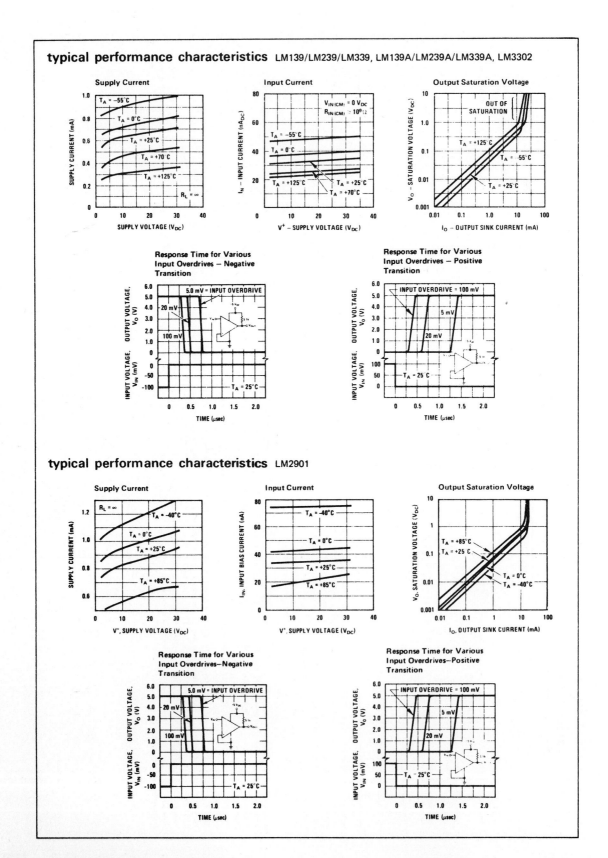

application hints

The LM139 series are high gain, wide bandwidth devices which, like most comparators, can easily oscillate if the output lead is inadvertently allowed to capacitively couple to the inputs via stray capacitance. This shows up only during the output voltage transition intervals as the comparator changes states. Power supply bypassing is not required to solve this problem. Standard PC board layout is helpful as it reduces stray input-output coupling. Reducing the input resistors to < 10 kΩ reduces the feedback signal levels and finally, adding even a small amount (1 to 10 mV) of positive feedback (hysteresis) causes such a rapid transition that oscillations due to stray feedback are not possible. Simply socketing the IC and attaching resistors to the pins will cause input-output oscillations during the small transition intervals unless hysteresis is used. If the input signal is a pulse waveform, with relatively fast rise and fall times, hysteresis is not required.

All pins of any unused comparators should be grounded.

The bias network of the LM139 series establishes a drain current which is independent of the magnitude of the power supply voltage over the range of from 2 V_{DC} to 30 V_{DC}.

It is usually unnecessary to use a bypass capacitor across the power supply line.

The differential input voltage may be larger than V^+ without damaging the device. Protection should be provided to prevent the input voltages from going negative more than -0.3 V_{DC} (at 25°C). An input clamp diode can be used as shown in the applications section.

The output of the LM139 series is the uncommitted collector of a grounded-emitter NPN output transistor. Many collectors can be tied together to provide an output OR'ing function. An output pull-up resistor can be connected to any available power supply voltage within the permitted supply voltage range and there is no restriction on this voltage due to the magnitude of the voltage which is applied to the V^+ terminal of the LM139A package. The output can also be used as a simple SPST switch to ground (when a pull-up resistor is not used). The amount of current which the output device can sink is limited by the drive available (which is independent of V^+) and the β of this device. When the maximum current limit is reached (approximately 16 mA), the output transistor will come out of saturation and the output voltage will rise very rapidly. The output saturation voltage is limited by the approximately 60Ω r_{sat} of the output transistor. The low offset voltage of the output transistor (1 mV) allows the output to clamp essentially to ground level for small load currents.

typical applications $(V^+ = 15\ V_{DC})$

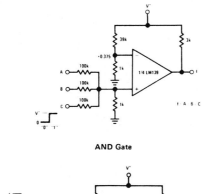

AND Gate

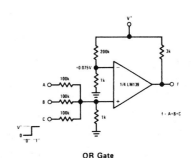

OR Gate

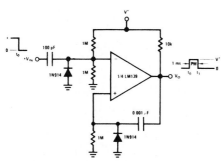

One-Shot Multivibrator

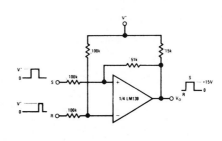

Bi-Stable Multivibrator

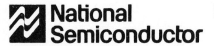

National Semiconductor

Industrial/Automotive/Functional Blocks/ Telecommunications

LM555/LM555C timer

general description

The LM555 is a highly stable device for generating accurate time delays or oscillation. Additional terminals are provided for triggering or resetting if desired. In the time delay mode of operation, the time is precisely controlled by one external resistor and capacitor. For astable operation as an oscillator, the free running frequency and duty cycle are accurately controlled with two external resistors and one capacitor. The circuit may be triggered and reset on falling waveforms, and the output circuit can source or sink up to 200 mA or drive TTL circuits.

features

- Direct replacement for SE555/NE555
- Timing from microseconds through hours
- Operates in both astable and monostable modes

- Adjustable duty cycle
- Output can source or sink 200 mA
- Output and supply TTL compatible
- Temperature stability better than 0.005% per °C
- Normally on and normally off output

applications

- Precision timing
- Pulse generation
- Sequential timing
- Time delay generation
- Pulse width modulation
- Pulse position modulation
- Linear ramp generator

---

schematic diagram

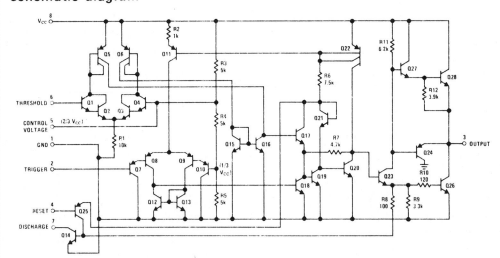

connection diagrams

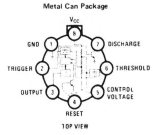

Metal Can Package

TOP VIEW

Order Number LM555H, LM555CH
See NS Package H08C

Dual-In-Line Package

TOP VIEW
Order Number LM555CN
See NS Package N08B
Order Number LM555J or LM555CJ
See NS Package J08A

absolute maximum ratings

Supply Voltage	+18V
Power Dissipation (Note 1)	600 mW
Operating Temperature Ranges	
LM555C	0°C to $+70^\circ$C
LM555	-55°C to $+125^\circ$C
Storage Temperature Range	-65°C to $+150^\circ$C
Lead Temperature (Soldering, 10 seconds)	300°C

electrical characteristics ($T_A = 25^\circ$C, V_{CC} = +5V to +15V, unless otherwise specified)

PARAMETER	CONDITIONS	LM555 MIN	LM555 TYP	LM555 MAX	LM555C MIN	LM555C TYP	LM555C MAX	UNITS
Supply Voltage		4.5		18	4.5		16	V
Supply Current	V_{CC} = 5V, $R_L = \infty$		3	5		3	6	mA
	V_{CC} = 15V, $R_L = \infty$ (Low State) (Note 2)		10	12		10	15	mA
Timing Error, Monostable								
Initial Accuracy			0.5	2		1		%
Drift with Temperature	R_A, R_B = 1k to 100 k, C = 0.1μF, (Note 3)		30			50		ppm/$^\circ$C
Accuracy over Temperature			1.5	3.0		1.5		%
Drift with Supply			0.05	0.2		0.1		%/V
Timing Error, Astable								
Initial Accuracy			1.5	5		2.25	7	%
Drift with Temperature			90			150		ppm/$^\circ$C
Accuracy over Temperature			2.5			3.0		%
Drift with Supply			0.15	0.2		0.30	0.5	%/V
Threshold Voltage			0.667			0.667		x V_{CC}
Trigger Voltage	V_{CC} = 15V	4.8	5	5.2		5		V
	V_{CC} = 5V	1.45	1.67	1.9		1.67		V
Trigger Current			0.01	0.5		0.5	0.9	μA
Reset Voltage		0.4	0.5	1	0.4	0.5	1	V
Reset Current			0.1	0.4		0.1	0.4	mA
Threshold Current	(Note 4)		0.1	0.25		0.1	0.25	μA
Control Voltage Level	V_{CC} = 15V	9.6	10	10.4	9	10	11	V
	V_{CC} = 5V	2.9	3.33	3.8	2.6	3.33	4	V
Pin 7 Leakage Output High			1	100		1	100	nA
Pin 7 Sat (Note 5)								
Output Low	V_{CC} = 15V, I_7 = 15 mA		150			180		mV
Output Low	V_{CC} = 4.5V, I_7 = 4.5 mA		70	100		80	200	mV
Output Voltage Drop (Low)	V_{CC} = 15V							
	I_{SINK} = 10 mA		0.1	0.15		0.1	0.25	V
	I_{SINK} = 50 mA		0.4	0.5		0.4	0.75	V
	I_{SINK} = 100 mA		2	2.2		2	2.5	V
	I_{SINK} = 200 mA		2.5			2.5		V
	V_{CC} = 5V							
	I_{SINK} = 8 mA		0.1	0.25				V
	I_{SINK} = 5 mA					0.25	0.35	V
Output Voltage Drop (High)	I_{SOURCE} = 200 mA, V_{CC} = 15V		12.5			12.5		V
	I_{SOURCE} = 100 mA, V_{CC} = 15V	13	13.3		12.75	13.3		V
	V_{CC} = 5V	3	3.3		2.75	3.3		V
Rise Time of Output			100			100		ns
Fall Time of Output			100			100		ns

Note 1: For operating at elevated temperatures the device must be derated based on a +150°C maximum junction temperature and a thermal resistance of +45°C/W junction to case for TO-5 and +150°C/W junction to ambient for both packages.
Note 2: Supply current when output high typically 1 mA less at V_{CC} = 5V.
Note 3: Tested at V_{CC} = 5V and V_{CC} = 15V.
Note 4: This will determine the maximum value of $R_A + R_B$ for 15V operation. The maximum total ($R_A + R_B$) is 20 MΩ.
Note 5: No protection against excessive pin 7 current is necessary providing the package dissipation rating will not be exceeded.

typical performance characteristics

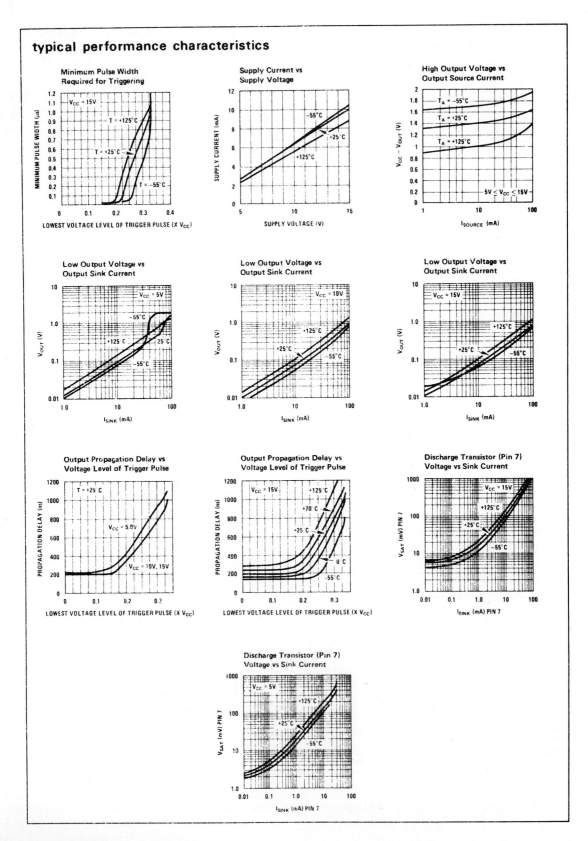

applications information

MONOSTABLE OPERATION

In this mode of operation, the timer functions as a one-shot (*Figure 1*). The external capacitor is initially held discharged by a transistor inside the timer. Upon application of a negative trigger pulse of less than 1/3 V_{CC} to pin 2, the flip-flop is set which both releases the short circuit across the capacitor and drives the output high.

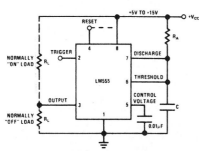

FIGURE 1. Monostable

The voltage across the capacitor then increases exponentially for a period of t = 1.1 R_AC, at the end of which time the voltage equals 2/3 V_{CC}. The comparator then resets the flip-flop which in turn discharges the capacitor and drives the output to its low state. *Figure 2* shows the waveforms generated in this mode of operation. Since the charge and the threshold level of the comparator are both directly proportional to supply voltage, the timing internal is independent of supply.

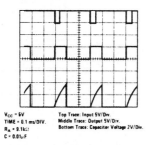

V_{CC} = 5V
TIME = 0.1 ms/DIV.
R_A = 9.1kΩ
C = 0.01µF

Top Trace: Input 5V/Div.
Middle Trace: Output 5V/Div.
Bottom Trace: Capacitor Voltage 2V/Div.

FIGURE 2. Monostable Waveforms

During the timing cycle when the output is high, the further application of a trigger pulse will not effect the circuit. However the circuit can be reset during this time by the application of a negative pulse to the reset terminal (pin 4). The output will then remain in the low state until a trigger pulse is again applied.

When the reset function is not in use, it is recommended that it be connected to V_{CC} to avoid any possibility of false triggering.

Figure 3 is a nomograph for easy determination of R, C values for various time delays.

ASTABLE OPERATION

If the circuit is connected as shown in *Figure 4* (pins 2 and 6 connected) it will trigger itself and free run as a

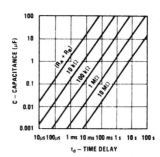

FIGURE 3. Time Delay

multivibrator. The external capacitor charges through R_A + R_B and discharges through R_B. Thus the duty cycle may be precisely set by the ratio of these two resistors.

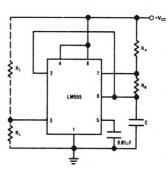

FIGURE 4. Astable

In this mode of operation, the capacitor charges and discharges between 1/3 V_{CC} and 2/3 V_{CC}. As in the triggered mode, the charge and discharge times, and therefore the frequency are independent of the supply voltage.

Figure 5 shows the waveforms generated in this mode of operation.

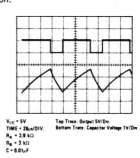

V_{CC} = 5V
TIME = 20µs/DIV.
R_A = 3.9 kΩ
R_B = 3 kΩ
C = 0.01µF

Top Trace: Output 5V/Div.
Bottom Trace: Capacitor Voltage 1V/Div.

FIGURE 5. Astable Waveforms

The charge time (output high) is given by:
$$t_1 = 0.693 (R_A + R_B) C$$

And the discharge time (output low) by:
$$t_2 = 0.693 (R_B) C$$

Thus the total period is:
$$T = t_1 + t_2 = 0.693 (R_A + 2R_B) C$$

applications information (con't)

The frequency of oscillation is:

$$f = \frac{1}{T} = \frac{1.44}{(R_A + 2R_B)C}$$

Figure 6 may be used for quick determination of these RC values.

The duty cycle is:

$$D = \frac{R_B}{R_A + 2R_B}$$

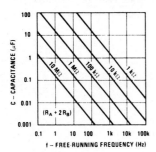

FIGURE 6. Free Running Frequency

FREQUENCY DIVIDER

The monostable circuit of *Figure 1* can be used as a frequency divider by adjusting the length of the timing cycle. *Figure 7* shows the waveforms generated in a divide by three circuit.

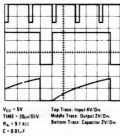

V_CC = 5V   Top Trace: Input 4V/Div.
TIME = 20μs/DIV.   Middle Trace: Output 2V/Div.
R_A = 9.1 kΩ   Bottom Trace: Capacitor 2V/Div.
C = 0.01μF

FIGURE 7. Frequency Divider

PULSE WIDTH MODULATOR

When the timer is connected in the monostable mode and triggered with a continuous pulse train, the output pulse width can be modulated by a signal applied to pin 5. *Figure 8* shows the circuit, and in *Figure 9* are some waveform examples.

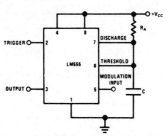

FIGURE 8. Pulse Width Modulator

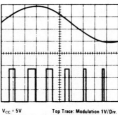

V_CC = 5V   Top Trace: Modulation 1V/Div.
TIME = 0.2 ms/DIV.   Bottom Trace: Output 2V/Div.
R_A = 9.1 kΩ
C = 0.01μF

FIGURE 9. Pulse Width Modulator

PULSE POSITION MODULATOR

This application uses the timer connected for astable operation, as in *Figure 10*, with a modulating signal again applied to the control voltage terminal. The pulse position varies with the modulating signal, since the threshold voltage and hence the time delay is varied. *Figure 11* shows the waveforms generated for a triangle wave modulation signal.

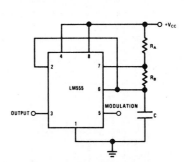

FIGURE 10. Pulse Position Modulator

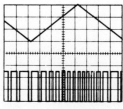

V_CC = 5V   Top Trace: Modulation Input 1V/Div.
TIME = 0.1 ms/DIV.   Bottom Trace: Output 2V/Div.
R_A = 3.9 kΩ
R_B = 3 kΩ
C = 0.01μF

FIGURE 11. Pulse Position Modulator

LINEAR RAMP

When the pullup resistor, R_A, in the monostable circuit is replaced by a constant current source, a linear ramp is

applications information (con't)

generated. *Figure 12* shows a circuit configuration that will perform this function.

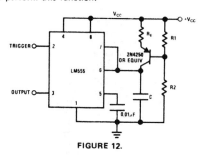

FIGURE 12.

Figure 13 shows waveforms generated by the linear ramp.

The time interval is given by:

$$T = \frac{2/3\ V_{CC}\ R_E\ (R_1 + R_2)\ C}{R_1\ V_{CC} - V_{BE}\ (R_1 + R_2)}$$

$$V_{BE} \simeq 0.6V$$

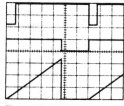

V_{CC} = 5V   Top Trace: Input 3V/Div.
TIME = 20μs/DIV.   Middle Trace: Output 5V/Div.
R_1 = 47 kΩ   Bottom Trace: Capacitor Voltage 1V/Div.
R_2 = 100 kΩ
R_E = 2.7 kΩ
C = 0.01μF

FIGURE 13. Linear Ramp

50% DUTY CYCLE OSCILLATOR

For a 50% duty cycle, the resistors R_A and R_B may be connected as in *Figure 14*. The time period for the out-

put high is the same as previous, t_1 = 0.693 R_A C. For the output low it is t_2 =

$$[(R_A\ R_B)/(R_A + R_B)]\ CLn \left[\frac{R_B - 2R_A}{2R_B - R_A}\right]$$

Thus the frequency of oscillation is $f = \dfrac{1}{t_1 + t_2}$

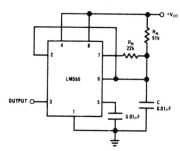

FIGURE 14. 50% Duty Cycle Oscillator

Note that this circuit will not oscillate if R_B is greater than 1/2 R_A because the junction of R_A and R_B cannot bring pin 2 down to 1/3 V_{CC} and trigger the lower comparator.

ADDITIONAL INFORMATION

Adequate power supply bypassing is necessary to protect associated circuitry. Minimum recommended is 0.1μF in parallel with 1μF electrolytic.

Lower comparator storage time can be as long as 10μs when pin 2 is driven fully to ground for triggering. This limits the monostable pulse width to 10μs minimum.

Delay time reset to output is 0.47μs typical. Minimum reset pulse width must be 0.3μs, typical.

Pin 7 current switches within 30 ns of the output (pin 3) voltage.

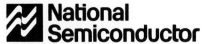 **National
Semiconductor**

**Industrial/Automotive/Functional
Blocks/ Telecommunications**

LM556/LM556C dual timer
general description

The LM556 Dual timing circuit is a highly stable controller capable of producing accurate time delays or oscillation. The 556 is a dual 555. Timing is provided by an external resistor and capacitor for each timing function. The two timers operate independently of each other sharing only V_{CC} and ground. The circuits may be triggered and reset on falling waveforms. The output structures may sink or source 200 mA.

- Adjustable duty cycle
- Output can source or sink 200 mA
- Output and supply TTL compatible
- Temperature stability better than 0.005% per $^{\circ}$C
- Normally on and normally off output

applications
- Precision timing
- Pulse generation
- Sequential timing
- Time delay generation
- Pulse width modulation
- Pulse position modulation
- Linear ramp generator

features
- Direct replacement for SE556/NE556
- Timing from microseconds through hours
- Operates in both astable and monostable modes
- Replaces two 555 timers

schematic diagram

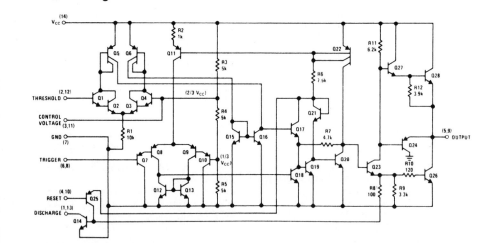

connection diagram

Dual-In-Line Package

Order Number LM556CN
See NS Package N14A

Order Number LM556J or LM556CJ
See NS Package J14A

Courtesy of National Semiconductor Corporation

absolute maximum ratings

Supply Voltage	+18V
Power Dissipation (Note 1)	600 mW
Operating Temperature Ranges	
LM556C	$0°C$ to $+70°C$
LM556	$-55°C$ to $+125°C$
Storage Temperature Range	$-65°C$ to $+150°C$
Lead Temperature (Soldering, 10 seconds)	$300°C$

electrical characteristics ($T_A = 25°C$, $V_{CC} = +5V$ to $+15V$, unless otherwise specified)

PARAMETER	CONDITIONS	LM556 MIN	LM556 TYP	LM556 MAX	LM556C MIN	LM556C TYP	LM556C MAX	UNITS
Supply Voltage		4.5		18	4.5		16	V
Supply Current	$V_{CC} = 5V$, $R_L = \infty$		3	5		3	6	mA
(Each Timer Section)	$V_{CC} = 15V$, $R_L = \infty$		10	11		10	14	mA
	(Low State) (Note 2)							
Timing Error, Monostable								
Initial Accuracy			0.5	1.5		0.75	5.0	%
Drift With Temperature	R_A, R_B = 1k to 100k, C = 0.1μF,		30			50		ppm/°C
	(Note 3)							
Accuracy Over Temperature			1.5	5		1.5		%
Drift with Supply			0.05	0.2		0.1	0.4	%/V
Timing Error, Astable								
Initial Accuracy			1.5			2.25	7	%
Drift With Temperature			90			150		ppm/°C
Accuracy Over Temperature			2.5			3.0		%
Drift With Supply			0.15	0.2		0.30		%/V
Trigger Voltage	$V_{CC} = 15V$	4.8	5	5.2	4.5	5	0.5	V
	$V_{CC} = 5V$	1.45	1.67	1.9	1.25	1.67	2.0	V
Trigger Current			0.1	0.5		0.2	1.0	μA
Reset Voltage	(Note 4)	0.4	0.5	1	0.4	0.5	1	V
Reset Current			0.1	0.4		0.1	0.6	mA
Threshold Current	(Note 5)		0.03	0.1		0.03	0.1	μA
Control Voltage Level And	$V_{CC} = 15V$	9.6	10	10.4	9	10	11	V
Threshold Voltage	$V_{CC} = 5V$	2.9	3.33	3.8	2.6	3.33	4	V
Pin 1, 13 Leakage Output High			1	100		1	100	nA
Pin 1, 13 Sat	(Note 6)							
Output Low	$V_{CC} = 15V$, I = 15 mA		150	240		180	300	mV
Output Low	$V_{CC} = 4.5V$, I = 4.5 mA		70	100		80	200	mV
Output Voltage Drop (Low)	$V_{CC} = 15V$							
	$I_{SINK} = 10$ mA		0.1	0.15		0.1	0.25	V
	$I_{SINK} = 50$ mA		0.4	0.5		0.4	0.75	V
	$I_{SINK} = 100$ mA		2	2.25		2	2.75	V
	$I_{SINK} = 200$ mA		2.5			2.5		V
	$V_{CC} = 5V$							
	$I_{SINK} = 8$ mA		0.1	0.25				V
	$I_{SINK} = 5$ mA					0.25	0.35	V
Output Voltage Drop (High)	$I_{SOURCE} = 200$ mA, $V_{CC} = 15V$		12.5			12.5		V
	$I_{SOURCE} = 100$ mA, $V_{CC} = 15V$	13	13.3		12.75	13.3		V
	$V_{CC} = 5V$	3	3.3		2.75	3.3		V
Rise Time of Output			100			100		ns
Fall Time of Output			100			100		ns
Matching Characteristics	(Note 7)							
Initial Timing Accuracy			0.05	0.2		0.1	2.0	%
Timing Drift With Temperature			±10			±10		ppm/°C
Drift With Supply Voltage			0.1	0.2		0.2	0.5	%/V

Note 1: For operating at elevated temperatures the device must be derated based on a +150°C maximum junction temperature and a thermal resistance of +150°C/W junction to ambient for both packages.

Note 2: Supply current when output high typically 1 mA less at $V_{CC} = 5V$.

Note 3: Tested at $V_{CC} = 5V$ and $V_{CC} = 15V$.

Note 4: As reset voltage lowers, timing is inhibited and then the output goes low.

Note 5: This will determine the maximum value of $R_A + R_B$ for 15V operation. The maximum total ($R_A + R_B$) is 20 MΩ.

Note 6: No protection against excessive pin 1, 13 current is necessary providing the package dissipation rating will not be exceeded.

Note 7: Matching characteristics refer to the difference between performance characteristics of each timer section.

QUADRUPLE 2-INPUT POSITIVE NAND GATE

S5400
N7400

S5400–A,F,W • N7400–A,F

DIGITAL 54/74 TTL SERIES

SCHEMATIC (each gate)

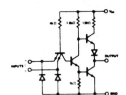

A,F PACKAGE

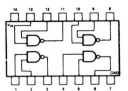

RECOMMENDED OPERATING CONDITIONS

	MIN	NOM	MAX	UNIT
Supply Voltage V_{CC}: S5400 Circuits	4.5	5	5.5	V
N7400 Circuits	4.75	5	5.25	V
Normalized Fan-Out from each Output, N			10	
Operating Free-Air Temperature Range, T_A: S5400 Circuits	-55	25	125	°C
N7400 Circuits	0	25	70	°C

ELECTRICAL CHARACTERISTICS (over recommended operating free-air temperature range unless otherwise noted)

PARAMETER		TEST CONDITIONS*		MIN	TYP**	MAX	UNIT
$V_{in(1)}$	Logical 1 input voltage required at both input terminals to ensure logical 0 level at output	V_{CC} = MIN		2			V
$V_{in(0)}$	Logical 0 input voltage required at either input terminal to ensure logical 1 level at output	V_{CC} = MIN				0.8	V
$V_{out(1)}$	Logical 1 output voltage	V_{CC} = MIN, I_{load} = −400µA	V_{in} = 0.8V,	2.4	3.3		V
$V_{out(0)}$	Logical 0 output voltage	V_{CC} = MIN, I_{sink} = 16mA	V_{in} = 2V,		0.22	0.4	V
$I_{in(0)}$	Logical 0 level input current (each input)	V_{CC} = MAX,	V_{in} = 0.4V			−1.6	mA
$I_{in(1)}$	Logical 1 level input current (each input)	V_{CC} = MAX, V_{CC} = MAX,	V_{in} = 2.4V V_{in} = 5.5V			40 1	µA mA
I_{OS}	Short circuit output current†	V_{CC} = MAX	S5400 N7400	−20 −18		−55 −55	mA

PARAMETER		TEST CONDITIONS*		MIN	TYP**	MAX	UNIT
$I_{CC(0)}$	Logical 0 level supply current	V_{CC} = MAX,	V_{in} = 5V		12	22	mA
$I_{CC(1)}$	Logical 1 level supply current	V_{CC} = MAX,	V_{in} = 0		4	8	mA

SWITCHING CHARACTERISTICS, V_{CC} = 5V, T_A = 25°C, N = 10

PARAMETER		TEST CONDITIONS		MIN	TYP	MAX	UNIT
$t_{pd(0)}$	Propagation delay time to logical 0 level	C_L = 15pF,	R_L = 400Ω		7	15	ns
$t_{pd(1)}$	Propagation delay time to logical 1 level	C_L = 15pF,	R_L = 400Ω		11	22	ns

* For conditions shown as MIN or MAX, use the appropriate value specified under recommended operating conditions for the applicable device type.
** All typical values are at V_{CC} = 5V, T_A = 25°C
† Not more than one output should be shorted at a time.

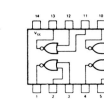

SCHEMATIC (each gate)

A,F PACKAGE

RECOMMENDED OPERATING CONDITIONS

PARAMETER		MIN	NOM	MAX	UNIT
Supply Voltage V_{CC}:	S5402 Circuits	4.5	5	5.5	V
	N7402 Circuits	4.75	5	5.25	V
Normalized Fan-Out from each Output, N				10	
Operating Free-Air Temperature Range, T_A:	S5402 Circuits	-55	25	125	°C
	N7402 Circuits	0	25	70	°C

ELECTRICAL CHARACTERISTICS (over recommended operating free-air temperature range unless otherwise noted)

PARAMETER		TEST CONDITIONS*		MIN	TYP**	MAX	UNIT
$V_{in(1)}$	Logical 1 input voltage required at either input terminal to ensure logical 0 level at output	V_{CC} = MIN		2			V
$V_{in(0)}$	Logical 0 input voltage required at both input terminals to ensure logical 1 level at output	V_{CC} = MIN				0.8	V
$V_{out(1)}$	Logical 1 output voltage	V_{CC} = MIN, I_{load} = −400μA	V_{in} = 0.8V	2.4	3.3		V
$V_{out(0)}$	Logical 0 output voltage	V_{CC} = MIN, I_{sink} = 16mA	V_{in} = 2V,		0.22	0.4	V
$I_{in(0)}$	Logical 0 level input current (each input)	V_{CC} = MAX,	V_{in} = 0.4V			−1.6	mA
$I_{in(1)}$	Logical 1 level input current (each input)	V_{CC} = MAX,	V_{in} = 2.4V			40	μA
		V_{CC} = MAX,	V_{in} = 5.5V			1	mA
I_{OS}	Short circuit output Current†	V_{CC} = MAX	S5402	−20		−55	mA
			N7402	−18		−55	

PARAMETER		TEST CONDITIONS*		MIN	TYP	MAX	UNIT
$I_{CC(0)}$	Logical 0 level supply current	V_{CC} = MAX,	V_{in} = 5V		14	27	mA
$I_{CC(1)}$	Logical 1 level supply current	V_{CC} = MAX,	V_{in} = 0		8	16	mA

SWITCHING CHARACTERISTICS, V_{CC} = 5V, T_A = 25°C, N = 10

PARAMETER		TEST CONDITIONS		MIN	TYP	MAX	UNIT
t_{pd0}	Propagation delay time to logical 0 level	C_L = 15pF,	R_L = 400Ω		8	15	ns
t_{pd1}	Propagation delay time to logical 1 level	C_L = 15pF,	R_L = 400Ω		12	22	ns

* For conditions shown as MIN or MAX, use the appropriate value specified under recommended operating conditions for the applicable device type.

** All typical values are at V_{CC} = 5V, T_A = 25°C

† Not more than one output should be shorted at a time.

SCHEMATIC (each inverter)

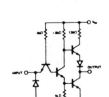

A,F PACKAGE

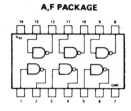

RECOMMENDED OPERATING CONDITIONS

	MIN	NOM	MAX	UNIT
Supply Voltage V_{CC}: S5404 Circuits	4.5	5	5.5	V
N7404 Circuits	4.75	5	5.25	V
Normalized Fan-Out from Output, N			10	
Operating Free-Air Temperature Range, T_A: S5404 Circuits	-55	25	125	°C
N7404 Circuits	0	25	70	°C

ELECTRICAL CHARACTERISTICS (over recommended operating free-air temperature range unless otherwise noted)

PARAMETER		TEST CONDITIONS*			MIN	TYP**	MAX	UNIT
$V_{in(1)}$	Logical 1 input voltage required at input terminal to ensure logical 0 level at output	V_{CC} = MIN			2			V
$V_{in(0)}$	Logical 0 input voltage required at any input terminal to ensure logical 1 level at output	V_{CC} = MIN					0.8	V
$V_{out(1)}$	Logical 1 output voltage	V_{CC} = MIN, I_{load} = -400μA	V_{in} = 0.8V,		2.4	3.3		V
$V_{out(0)}$	Logical 0 output voltage	V_{CC} = MIN, I_{sink} = 16mA	V_{in} = 2V,			0.22	0.4	V
$I_{in(0)}$	Logical 0 level input current (each input)	V_{CC} = MAX,	V_{in} = 0.4V				-1.6	mA
$I_{in(1)}$	Logical 1 level input current	V_{CC} = MAX,	V_{in} = 2.4V				40	μA
		V_{CC} = MAX,	V_{in} = 5.5V				1	mA
I_{OS}	Short circuit output current†	V_{CC} = MAX		S5404	-20		-55	mA
				N7404	-18		-55	

PARAMETER		TEST CONDITIONS*		MIN	TYP	MAX	UNIT
$I_{CC(0)}$	Logical 0 level supply current	V_{CC} = MAX,	V_{in} = 5V		18	33	mA
$I_{CC(1)}$	Logical 1 level supply current	V_{CC} = MAX,	V_{in} = 0		6	12	mA

SWITCHING CHARACTERISTICS, V_{CC} = 5V, T_A = 25°C, N = 10

PARAMETER		TEST CONDITIONS		MIN	TYP	MAX	UNIT
t_{pd0}	Propagation delay time to logical 0 level	C_L = 15pF,	R_L = 400Ω		8	15	ns
t_{pd1}	Propagation delay time to logical 1 level	C_L = 15pF,	R_L = 400Ω		12	22	ns

* For conditions shown as MIN or MAX, use the appropriate value specified under recommended operating conditions for the applicable device type.
** All typical values are at V_{CC} = 5V, T_A = 25°C.
† Not more than one output should be shorted at a time.

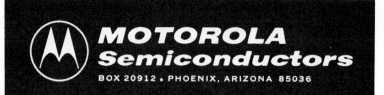

MOTOROLA Semiconductors
BOX 20912 • PHOENIX, ARIZONA 85036

MC1595L
MC1495L

Specifications and Applications Information

WIDEBAND MONOLITHIC FOUR-QUADRANT MULTIPLIER

. . . designed for uses where the output is a linear product of two input voltages. Maximum versatility is assured by allowing the user to select the level shift method. Typical applications include: multiply, divide*, square root*, mean square*, phase detector, frequency doubler, balanced modulator/demodulator, electronic gain control.

*When used with an operational amplifier.

- Wide Bandwidth

- Excellent Linearity — 1% max Error on X-Input, 2% max Error on Y-Input — MC1595L

- Excellent Linearity — 2% max Error on X-Input, 4% max Error on Y-Input — MC1495L

- Adjustable Scale Factor, K

- Excellent Temperature Stability

- Wide Input Voltage Range — ± 10 Volts

- ± 15 Volt Operation

LINEAR FOUR-QUADRANT MULTIPLIER

SILICON MONOLITHIC INTEGRATED CIRCUIT

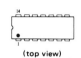

(top view)

CERAMIC PACKAGE
CASE 632
TO-116

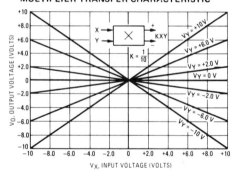

FIGURE 1 – FOUR-QUADRANT MULTIPLIER TRANSFER CHARACTERISTIC

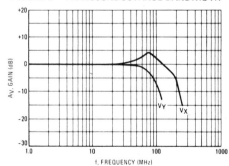

FIGURE 2 – TRANSCONDUCTANCE BANDWIDTH

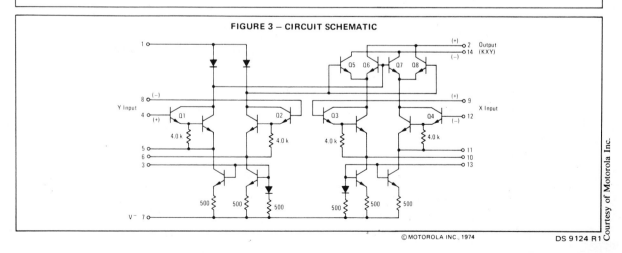

FIGURE 3 – CIRCUIT SCHEMATIC

© MOTOROLA INC., 1974

DS 9124 R1

ELECTRICAL CHARACTERISTICS (V^+ = +32V, V^- = -15 V, T_A = +25°C, I_3 = I_{13} = 1 mA, R_X = R_Y = 15 kΩ, R_L = 11 kΩ unless otherwise noted)

Characteristic		Figure	Symbol	Min	Typ	Max	Unit
Linearity: Output Error in Percent of Full Scale: T_A = +25°C		5					%
$-10 < V_X < +10$ ($V_Y = \pm10$ V)	MC1495		E_{RX}	–	± 1.0	± 2.0	
	MC1595			–	± 0.5	± 1.0	
$-10 < V_Y < +10$ ($V_X = \pm10$ V)	MC1495		E_{RY}	–	± 2.0	± 4.0	
	MC1595			–	± 1.0	± 2.0	
T_A = 0 to +70°C	MC1495						
$-10 < V_X < +10$ ($V_Y = \pm10$ V)			E_{RX}	–	± 1.5	–	
$-10 < V_Y < +10$ ($V_X = \pm10$ V)			E_{RY}	–	± 3.0	–	
T_A = -55°C to +125°C	MC1595						
$-10 < V_X < +10$ ($V_Y = \pm10$ V)			E_{RX}	–	+ 0.75	–	
$-10 < V_Y < +10$ ($V_X = \pm10$ V)			E_{RY}	–	± 1.50	–	
Squaring Mode Error: Accuracy in Percent of Full Scale After Offset and Scale Factor Adjustment		5	E_{SQ}				%
T_A = +25°C	MC1495			–	± 0.75	–	
	MC1595			–	± 0.5	–	
T_A = 0 to +70°C	MC1495			–	± 1.0	–	
T_A = -55°C to +125°C	MC1595			–	± 0.75	–	
Scale Factor (Adjustable) ($K = \dfrac{2R_L}{I_3 R_X R_Y}$)		–	K	–	0.1	–	–
Input Resistance (f = 20 Hz)	MC1495	7	R_{INX}	–	20	–	MegOhms
	MC1595				35		
	MC1495		R_{INY}		20		
	MC1595				35		
Differential Output Resistance (f = 20 Hz)		8	R_o		300	–	k Ohms
Input Bias Current $I_{bx} = \dfrac{(I_9 + I_{12})}{2}$, $I_{by} = \dfrac{(I_4 + I_8)}{2}$	MC1495	6	I_{bx}		2.0	12	μA
	MC1595				2.0	8.0	
	MC1495		I_{by}		2.0	12	
	MC1595			–	2.0	8.0	
Input Offset Current $|I_9 - I_{12}|$	MC1495	6	$|I_{iox}|$	–	0.4	2.0	μA
	MC1595				0.2	1.0	
$|I_4 - I_8|$	MC1495		$|I_{ioy}|$	–	0.4	2.0	
	MC1595				0.2	1.0	
Average Temperature Coefficient of Input Offset Current		6	$|TC_{lio}|$				nA/°C
(T_A = 0 to +70°C)	MC1495				2.0	–	
(T_A = -55°C to +125°C)	MC1595				2.0	–	
Output Offset Current $|I_{14} - I_2|$	MC1495	6	$|I_{oo}|$		20	100	μA
	MC1595				10	50	
Average Temperature Coefficient of Output Offset Current		6	$|TC_{loo}|$				nA/°C
(T_A = 0 to +70°C)	MC1495				20	–	
(T_A = -55°C to +125°C)	MC1595				20	–	
Frequency Response							
3.0 dB Bandwidth, R_L = 11 kΩ		9,10	BW3dB		3.0	–	MHz
3.0 dB Bandwidth, R_L = 50 Ω (Transconductance Bandwidth)			$T_{BW3 dB}$		80	–	MHz
3° Relative Phase Shift Between V_X and V_Y			f_ϕ		750	–	kHz
1% Absolute Error Due to Input-Output Phase Shift			f_θ		30	–	kHz
Common Mode Input Swing (Either Input)	MC1495	11	CMV	±10.5	±12	–	Vdc
	MC1595			±11.5	±13	–	
Common Mode Gain (Either Input)	MC1495	11	A_{CM}	-40	-50	–	dB
	MC1595			-50	-60	–	
Common Mode Quiescent Output Voltage		12	V_{o1}	–	21	–	Vdc
			V_{o2}	–	21	–	
Differential Output Voltage Swing Capability		9	V_O	–	+14	–	V_{peak}
Power Supply Sensitivity		12	S^+	–	5.0	–	mV/V
			S^-		10		
Power Supply Current		12	I_7	–	6.0	7.0	mA
DC Power Dissipation		12	P_D	–	135	170	mW

MOTOROLA *Semiconductor Products Inc.*

MAXIMUM RATINGS (T_A = +25°C unless otherwise noted)

Rating	Symbol	Value	Unit
Applied Voltage (V_2-V_1, $V_{14}-V_1$, V_1-V_9, V_1-V_{12}, V_1-V_4, V_1-V_8, $V_{12}-V_7$, V_9-V_7, V_8-V_7, V_4-V_7)	$\triangle V$	30	Vdc
Differential Input Signal	$V_{12}-V_9$ V_4-V_8	$\pm(6+I_{13}R_X)$ $\pm(6+I_3R_Y)$	Vdc Vdc
Maximum Bias Current	I_3 I_{13}	10 10	mA
Power Dissipation (Package Limitation) Ceramic Package Derate above T_A = +25°C	P_D	750 5.0	mW mW/°C
Operating Temperature Range MC1495 MC1595	T_A	 0 to +70 −55 to +125	°C °C °C
Storage Temperature Range	T_{stg}	−65 to +150	°C

TEST CIRCUITS

FIGURE 4 — LINEARITY (USING NULL TECHNIQUE)

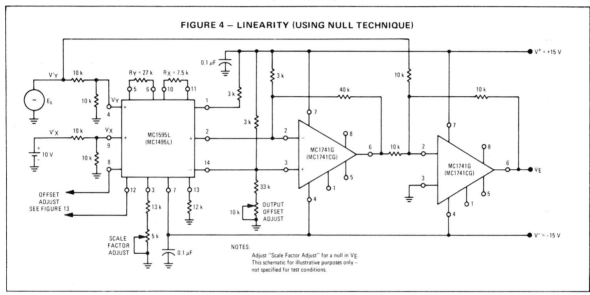

NOTES:
Adjust "Scale Factor Adjust" for a null in V_E.
This schematic for illustrative purposes only —
not specified for test conditions.

FIGURE 5 — LINEARITY (USING X-Y PLOTTER TECHNIQUE)

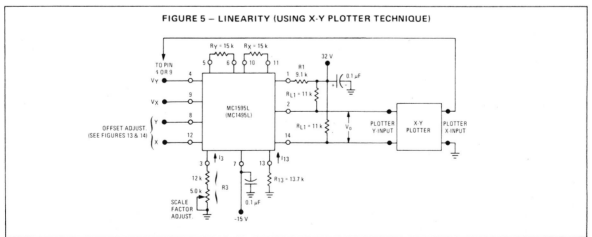

MOTOROLA *Semiconductor Products Inc.*

TEST CIRCUITS (continued)

FIGURE 6 – INPUT AND OUTPUT CURRENT

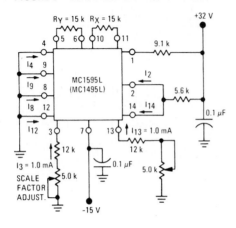

FIGURE 7 – INPUT RESISTANCE

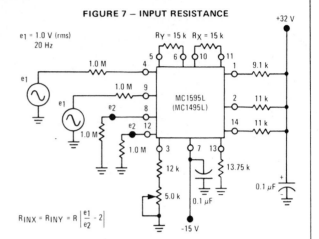

$$R_{INX} = R_{INY} = R \left| \frac{e1}{e2} - 2 \right|$$

FIGURE 8 – OUTPUT RESISTANCE

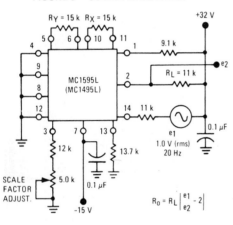

$$R_O = R_L \left| \frac{e1}{e2} - 2 \right|$$

FIGURE 9 – BANDWIDTH (R_L = 11 kΩ)

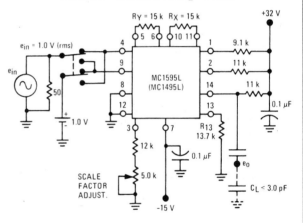

FIGURE 10 – BANDWIDTH (R_L = 50 Ω)

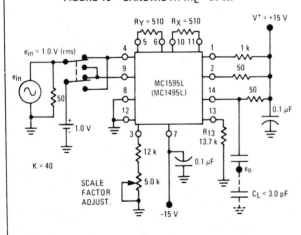

FIGURE 11 – COMMON-MODE GAIN and COMMON-MODE INPUT SWING

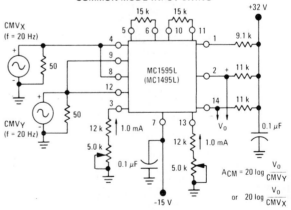

$$A_{CM} = 20 \log \frac{V_0}{CMV_Y}$$

$$\text{or } 20 \log \frac{V_0}{CMV_X}$$

TEST CIRCUITS (continued)

FIGURE 12 — POWER SUPPLY SENSITIVITY

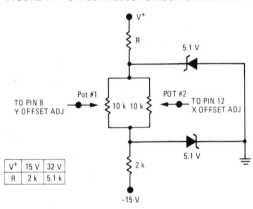

$$S^+ = \frac{|\Delta(V_{o1} - V_{o2})|}{\Delta V^+}$$

$$S^- = \frac{|\Delta(V_{o1} - V_{o2})|}{\Delta V^-}$$

FIGURE 13 — OFFSET ADJUST CIRCUIT

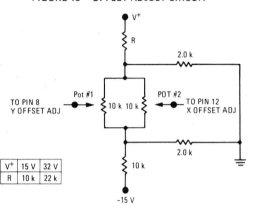

V+	15 V	32 V
R	10 k	22 k

FIGURE 14 — OFFSET ADJUST CIRCUIT (ALTERNATE)

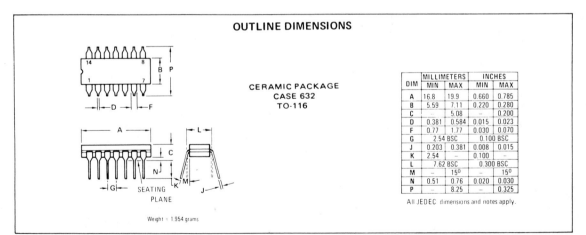

V+	15 V	32 V
R	2 k	5.1 k

OUTLINE DIMENSIONS

CERAMIC PACKAGE
CASE 632
TO-116

SEATING PLANE

Weight = 1.954 grams

DIM	MILLIMETERS		INCHES	
	MIN	MAX	MIN	MAX
A	16.8	19.9	0.660	0.785
B	5.59	7.11	0.220	0.280
C	–	5.08	–	0.200
D	0.381	0.584	0.015	0.023
F	0.77	1.77	0.030	0.070
G	2.54 BSC		0.100 BSC	
J	0.203	0.381	0.008	0.015
K	2.54	–	0.100	–
L	7.62 BSC		0.300 BSC	
M	–	15°	–	15°
N	0.51	0.76	0.020	0.030
P	–	8.25	–	0.325

All JEDEC dimensions and notes apply.

Ⓜ MOTOROLA *Semiconductor Products Inc.*

TYPICAL CHARACTERISTICS

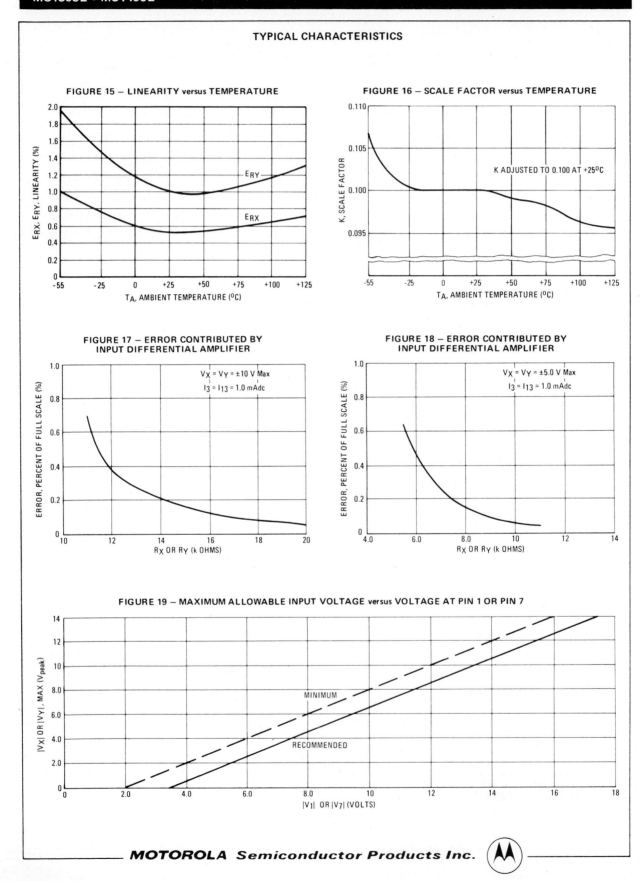

FIGURE 15 — LINEARITY versus TEMPERATURE

FIGURE 16 — SCALE FACTOR versus TEMPERATURE

FIGURE 17 — ERROR CONTRIBUTED BY INPUT DIFFERENTIAL AMPLIFIER

FIGURE 18 — ERROR CONTRIBUTED BY INPUT DIFFERENTIAL AMPLIFIER

FIGURE 19 — MAXIMUM ALLOWABLE INPUT VOLTAGE versus VOLTAGE AT PIN 1 OR PIN 7

MOTOROLA *Semiconductor Products Inc.*

OPERATION AND APPLICATIONS INFORMATION

1. Theory of Operation

The MC1595 (MC1495) is a monolithic, four-quadrant multiplier which operates on the principle of variable transconductance. The detailed theory of operation is covered in Application Note AN-489, Analysis and Basic Operation of the MC1595. The result of this analysis is that the differential output current of the multiplier is given by

$$I_A - I_B = \triangle I = \frac{2V_X V_Y}{R_X R_Y I_3}$$

where I_A and I_B are the currents into pins 14 and 2, respectively, and V_X and V_Y are the X and Y input voltages at the multiplier input terminals.

2. Design Considerations

2.1 General

The MC1595 (MC1495) permits the designer to tailor the multiplier to a specific application by proper selection of external components. External components may be selected to optimize a given parameter (e.g. bandwidth) which may in turn restrict another parameter (e.g. maximum output voltage swing). Each important parameter is discussed in detail in the following paragraphs.

2.1.1 Linearity, Output Error, E_{RX} or E_{RY}

Linearity error is defined as the maximum deviation of output voltage from a straight line transfer function. It is expressed as error in percent of full scale (see figure below).

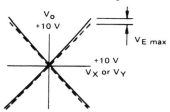

For example, if the maximum deviation, $V_{E(max)}$, is ±100 mV and the full scale output is 10 volts, then the percentage error is

$$E_R = \frac{V_{E(max)}}{V_{o(max)}} \times 100 = \frac{100 \times 10^{-3}}{10} \times 100 = \pm 1.0\%.$$

Linearity error may be measured by either of the following methods:

1. Using an X — Y plotter with the circuit shown in Figure 5, obtain plots for X and Y similar to the one shown above.
2. Use the circuit of Figure 4. This method nulls the level shifted output of the multiplier with the original input. The peak output of the null operational amplifier will be equal to the error voltage, $V_{E(max)}$.

One source of linearity error can arise from large signal non-linearity in the X and Y-input differential amplifiers. To avoid introducing error from this source, the emitter degeneration resistors R_X and R_Y must be chosen large enough so that non-linear base-emitter voltage variation can be ignored. Figures 17 and 18 show the error expected from this source as a function of the values of R_X and R_Y with an operating current of 1.0 mA in each side of the differential amplifiers (i.e., $I_3 = I_{13} = 1.0$ mA).

2.1.2 3 dB-Bandwidth and Phase Shift

Bandwidth is primarily determined by the load resistors and the stray multiplier output capacitance and/or the operational amplifier used to level shift the output. If wideband operation is desired, low value load resistors and/or a wideband operational amplifier should be used. Stray output capacitance will depend to a large extent on circuit layout.

Phase shift in the multiplier circuit results from two sources: phase shift common to both X and Y channels (due to the load resistor-output capacitance pole mentioned above) and relative phase shift between X and Y channels (due to differences in transadmittance in the X and Y channels). If the input to output phase shift is only 0.6°, the output product of two sine waves will exhibit a vector error of 1%. A 3° relative phase shift between V_X and V_Y results in a vector error of 5%.

2.1.3 Maximum Input Voltage

$V_{X(max)}$, $V_{Y(max)}$ maximum input voltages must be such that:

$$V_{X(max)} < I_{13} R_Y$$

$$V_{Y(max)} < I_3 R_Y.$$

Exceeding this value will drive one side of the input amplifier to "cutoff" and cause non-linear operation.

Currents I_3 and I_{13} are chosen at a convenient value (observing power dissipation limitation) between 0.5 mA and 2.0 mA, approximately 1.0 mA. Then R_X and R_Y can be determined by considering the input signal handling requirements.

For $V_{X(max)} = V_{Y(max)} = 10$ volts;

$$R_X = R_Y > \frac{10\text{ V}}{1.0\text{ mA}} = 10\text{ k}\Omega.$$

The equation $I_A - I_B = \dfrac{2V_X V_Y}{R_X R_Y I_3}$

is derived from $I_A - I_B = \dfrac{2V_X V_Y}{\left(R_X + \dfrac{2kT}{qI_{13}}\right)\left(R_Y + \dfrac{2kT}{qI_3}\right) I_3}$

with the assumption $R_X \gg \dfrac{2kT}{qI_{13}}$ and $R_Y \gg \dfrac{2kT}{qI_3}$

At $T_A = +25°C$ and $I_{13} = I_3 = 1$ mA,

$$\frac{2kT}{qI_{13}} = \frac{2kT}{qI_3} = 52\ \Omega.$$

Therefore, with $R_X = R_Y = 10$ kΩ the above assumption is valid. Reference to Figure 19 will indicate limitations of $V_{X(max)}$ or $V_{Y(max)}$ due to V_1 and V_7. Exceeding these limits will cause saturation or "cutoff" of the input transistors. See Step 4 of Section 3 (General Design Procedure) for further details.

2.1.4 Maximum Output Voltage Swing

The maximum output voltage swing is dependent upon the factors mentioned below and upon the particular circuit being considered.

For Figure 20 the maximum output swing is dependent upon V^+ for positive swing and upon the voltage at pin 1 for negative swing. The potential at pin 1 determines the quiescent level for transistors Q_5, Q_6, Q_7, and Q_8. This potential

 MOTOROLA *Semiconductor Products Inc.*

OPERATION AND APPLICATIONS INFORMATION (continued)

should be related so that negative swing at pins 2 or 14 does not saturate those transistors. See Section 3 for further information regarding selection of these potentials.

If an operational amplifier is used for level shift, as shown in Figure 21, the output swing (of the multiplier) is greatly reduced. See Section 3 for further details.

3. General Design Procedure

Selection of component values is best demonstrated by the following example: assume resistive dividers are used at the X and Y inputs to limit the maximum multiplier input to ±5.0 volts ($V_X = V_Y [max]$) for a ±10-volt input ($V_X' = V_Y' [max]$). (See Figure 21.) If an overall scale factor of 1/10 is desired, then

$$V_0 = \frac{V_X' V_Y'}{10} = \frac{(2V_X)(2V_Y)}{10} = 4/10 \ V_X V_Y .$$

Therefore, $K = 4/10$ for the multiplier (excluding the divider network).

Step 1. The first step is to select current I_3 and current I_{13}. There are no restrictions on the selection of either of these currents except the power dissipation of the device. I_3 and I_{13} will normally be one or two milliamperes. Further, I_3 does not have to be equal to I_{13}, and there is normally no need to make them different. For this example, let

$$I_3 = I_{13} = 1 \ mA.$$

To set currents I_3 and I_{13} to the desired value, it is only necessary to connect a resistor between pin 13 and ground, and between pin 3 and ground. From the schematic shown in Figure 3,

FIGURE 20 – BASIC MULTIPLIER

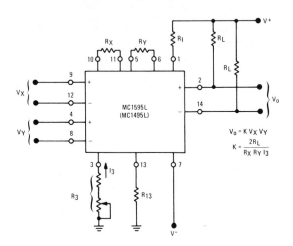

$$V_0 = K \ V_X \ V_Y$$
$$K = \frac{2R_L}{R_X \ R_Y \ I_3}$$

FIGURE 21 – MULTIPLIER WITH OP-AMPL. LEVEL SHIFT

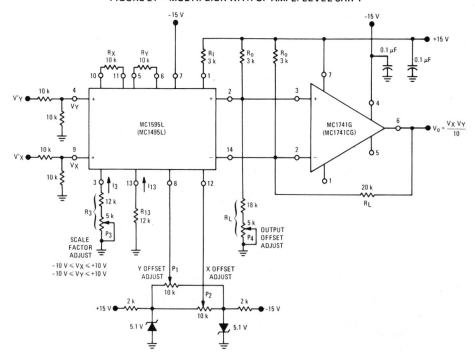

$$V_0 = \frac{V_X V_Y}{10}$$

MOTOROLA *Semiconductor Products Inc.*

OPERATION AND APPLICATIONS INFORMATION (continued)

it can be seen that the resistor values necessary are given by:

$$R_{13} + 500\ \Omega = \frac{|V^-| - 0.7\ V}{I_{13}}$$

$$R_3 + 500\ \Omega = \frac{|V^-| - 0.7\ V}{I_3}$$

Let $V^- = -15\ V$

Then $R_{13} + 500 = \dfrac{14.3\ V}{1\ mA}$ or $R_{13} = 13.8\ k\Omega$

Let $R_{13} = 12\ k\Omega$

Similarly, $R_3 = 13.8\ k\Omega$

Let $R_3 = 15\ k\Omega$

However, for applications which require an accurate scale factor, the adjustment of R_3 and consequently, I_3, offers a convenient method of making a final trim of the scale factor. For this reason, as shown in Figure 21, resistor R_3 is shown as a fixed resistor in series with a potentiometer.

For applications not requiring an exact scale factor (balanced modulator, frequency doubler, AGC amplifier, etc.), pins 3 and 13 can be connected together and a single resistor from pin 3 to ground can be used. In this case, the single resistor would have a value of one-half the above calculated value for R_{13}.

Step 2. The next step is to select R_X and R_Y. To insure that the input transistors will always be active, the following conditions should be met:

$$\frac{V_X}{R_X} < I_{13} \qquad \frac{V_Y}{R_Y} < I_3.$$

A good rule of thumb is to make $I_3 R_Y \geqslant 1.5\ V_{Y(max)}$ and $I_{13} R_X \geqslant 1.5\ V_{X(max)}$.

The larger the $I_3 R_Y$ and $I_{13} R_X$ product in relation to V_Y and V_X respectively, the more accurate the multiplier will be (see Figures 17 and 18).

Let $R_X = R_Y = 10\ k\Omega$

Then $I_3 R_Y = 10\ V$

$I_{13} R_X = 10\ V$

since $V_{X(max)} = V_{Y(max)} = 5.0$ volts the value of $R_X = R_Y = 10\ k\Omega$ is sufficient.

Step 3. Now that R_X, R_Y and I_3 have been chosen, R_L can be determined:

$$K = \frac{2R_L}{R_X R_Y I_3} = \frac{4}{10}$$

or $\dfrac{(2)\ (R_L)}{(10\ k)\ (10\ k)\ (1\ mA)} = \dfrac{4}{10}$

Thus $R_L = 20\ k\Omega$.

Step 4. To determine what power-supply voltage is necessary for this application, attention must be given to the circuit schematic shown in Figure 3. From the circuit schematic it can be seen that in order to maintain transistors Q_1, Q_2, Q_3 and Q_4 in an active region when the maximum input voltages are applied ($V_X' = V_Y' = 10\ V$ or $V_X = 5.0\ V$, $V_Y = 5.0\ V$), their respective collector voltage should be at least a few tenths of a volt higher than the maximum input voltage. It should also be noticed that the collector voltage of transistors Q_3 and Q_4 are at a potential which is two diode-drops below the voltage at pin 1. Thus, the voltage at pin 1 should be about two volts higher than the maximum input voltage. Therefore, to handle +5.0 volts at the inputs, the voltage at pin 1 must be at least +7.0 volts. Let $V_1 = 9.0\ Vdc$.

Since the current following into pin 1 is always equal to $2I_3$, the voltage at pin 1 can be set by placing a resistor, R_1 from pin 1 to the positive supply:

$$R_1 = \frac{V^+ - V_1}{2I_3}$$

Let $V^+ = +15\ V$

Then $R_1 = \dfrac{15\ V - 9\ V}{(2)\ (1\ mA)}$

$R_1 = 3\ k\Omega$.

Note that the voltage at the base of transistors Q_5, Q_6, Q_7 and Q_8 is one diode-drop below the voltage at pin 1. Thus, in order that these transistors stay active, the voltage at pins 2 and 14 should be approximately halfway between the voltage at pin 1 and the positive-supply voltage. For this example, the voltage at pins 2 and 14 should be approximately 11 volts.

Step 5. Level Shifting

For dc applications, such as the multiply, divide and square-root functions, it is usually desirable to convert the differential output to a single-ended output voltage referenced to ground. The circuit shown in Figure 22 performs this function. It can be shown that the output voltage of this circuit is given by:

$$V_o = (I_2 - I_{14})\ R_L$$

And since $I_A - I_B = I_2 - I_{14} = \dfrac{2I_X I_Y}{I_3} = \dfrac{2\ V_X V_Y}{I_3 R_X R_Y}$

Then $V_o = \dfrac{2R_L V_X' V_Y'}{4R_X R_X I_3}$ where $V_X' V_Y'$ is the voltage at the input to the voltage dividers.

FIGURE 22 — LEVEL SHIFT CIRCUIT

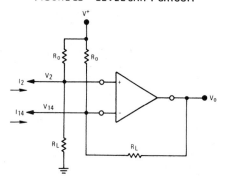

OPERATION AND APPLICATIONS INFORMATION (continued)

The choice of an operational amplifier for this application should have low bias currents, low offset current, and a high common-mode input voltage range as well as a high common-mode rejection ratio. The MC1556, and MC1741 operational amplifiers meet these requirements.

Referring to Figure 21, the level shift components will be determined. When $V_X = V_Y = 0$, the currents I_2 and I_{14} will be equal to I_{13}. In Step 3, R_L was found to be 20 kΩ and in Step 4, V_2 and V_{14} were found to be approximately 11 volts. From this information, R_o can be found easily from the following equation (neglecting the operational amplifiers bias current):

$$\frac{V_2}{R_L} + I_{13} = \frac{V^+ - V_2}{R_o}$$

And for this example, $\dfrac{11\ V}{20\ k\Omega} + 1\ mA = \dfrac{15\ V - 11\ V}{R_o}$

Solving for R_o, $R_o = 2.6\ k\Omega$

Thus, select $R_o = 3.0\ k\Omega$

For $R_o = 3.0\ k\Omega$, the voltage at pins 2 and 14 is calculated to be

$$V_2 = V_{14} = 10.4\ volts.$$

The linearity of this circuit (Figure 21) is likely to be as good or better than the circuit of Figure 5. Further improvements are possible as shown in Figure 23 where R_Y has been increased substantially to improve the Y linearity, and R_X decreased somewhat so as not to materially affect the X linearity, this avoids increasing R_L significantly in order to maintain a K of 0.1.

The versatility of the MC1595 (MC1495) allows the user to to optimize its performance for various input and output signal levels.

4. Offset and Scale Factor Adjustment

4.1 Offset Voltages

Within the monolithic multiplier (Figure 3) transistor base-emitter junctions are typically matched within 1 mV and resistors are typically matched within 2%. Even with this careful matching, an output error can occur. This output error is comprised of X-input offset voltage, Y-input offset voltage, and output-offset voltage. These errors can be adjusted to zero with the techniques shown in Figure 21. Offset terms can be shown analytically by the transfer function:

$$V_O = K(V_X \pm V_{IOX} \pm V_X\ off)(V_Y \pm V_{IOY} \pm V_Y\ off) \pm V_{oo} \quad (1)$$

Where K = scale factor
V_X = X input voltage
V_Y = Y input voltage
V_{IOX} = X input offset voltage
V_{IOY} = Y input offset voltage
$V_X\ off$ = X input offset adjust voltage
$V_Y\ off$ = Y input offset adjust voltage
V_{oo} = output offset voltage.

FIGURE 23 – MULTIPLIER WITH IMPROVED LINEARITY

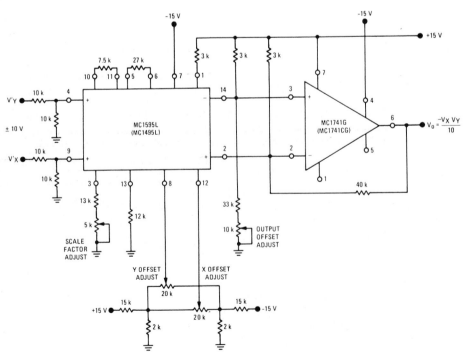

MOTOROLA *Semiconductor Products Inc.*

OPERATION AND APPLICATIONS INFORMATION (continued)

X, Y and Output Offset Voltages

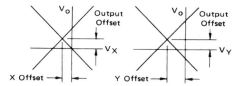

For most dc applications, all three offset adjust potentiometers (P_1, P_2, P_4) will be necessary. One or more offset adjust potentiometers can be eliminated for ac applications (See Figures 28, 29, 30, 31).

If well regulated supply voltages are available, the offset adjust circuit of Figure 13 is recommended. Otherwise, the circuit of Figure 14 will greatly reduce the sensitivity to power supply changes.

4.2 Scale Factor

The scale factor, K, is set by P_3 (Figure 21). P_3 varies I_3 which inversely controls the scale factor K. It should be noted that current I_3 is one-half the current through R_1. R_1 sets the bias level for Q_5, Q_6, Q_7, and Q_8 (See Figure 3). Therefore, to be sure that these devices remain active under all conditions of input and output swing, care should be exercised in adjusting P_3 over wide voltage ranges (see Section 3, General Design Procedure).

4.3 Adjustment Procedures

The following adjustment procedure should be used to null the offsets and set the scale factor for the multiply mode of operation. (See Figure 21)

1. X Input Offset
   (a) Connect oscillator (1 kHz, 5 Vpp sinewave) to the "Y" input (pin 4)
   (b) Connect "X" input (pin 9) to ground
   (c) Adjust X offset potentiometer, P_2, for an ac null at the output
2. Y Input Offset
   (a) Connect oscillator (1 kHz, 5 Vpp sinewave) to the "X" input (pin 9)
   (b) Connect "Y" input (pin 4) to ground
   (c) Adjust "Y" offset potentiometer, P_1, for an ac null at the output
3. Output Offset
   (a) Connect both "X" and "Y" inputs to ground
   (b) Adjust output offset potentiometer, P_4, until the output voltage V_o is zero volts dc
4. Scale Factor
   (a) Apply +10 Vdc to both the "X" and "Y" inputs
   (b) Adjust P_3 to achieve +10.00 V at the output.
5. Repeat steps 1 through 4 as necessary.

The ability to accurately adjust the MC1595 (MC1495) depends upon the characteristics of potentiometers P_1 through P_4. Multi-turn, infinite resolution potentiometers with low-temperature coefficients are recommended.

5. DC Applications

5.1 Multiply

The circuit shown in Figure 21 may be used to multiply signals from dc to 100 kHz. Input levels to the actual multiplier are 5.0 V (max). With resistive voltage dividers the maximum could be very large — however, for this application two-to-one dividers have been used so that the maximum input level is 10 V. The maximum output level has also been designed for 10 V (max).

5.2 Squaring Circuit

If the two inputs are tied together, the resultant function is squaring; that is $V_o = KV^2$ where K is the scale factor. Note that all error terms can be eliminated with only three adjustment potentiometers, thus eliminating one of the input offset adjustments. Procedures for nulling with adjustments are given as follows:

1. AC Procedure:
   (a) Connect oscillator (1 kHz, 15 Vpp) to input
   (b) Monitor output at 2 kHz with tuned voltmeter and adjust P_3 for desired gain (be sure to peak response of the voltmeter)
   (c) Tune voltmeter to 1 kHz and adjust P_1 for a minimum output voltage
   (d) Ground input and adjust P_4 (output offset) for zero volts dc output
   (e) Repeat steps a through d as necessary.
2. DC Procedure:
   (a) Set $V_X = V_Y = 0$ V and adjust P_4 (output offset potentiometer) such that $V_o = 0.0$ Vdc
   (b) Set $V_X = V_Y = 1.0$ V and adjust P_1 (Y input offset potentiometer) such that the output voltage is +0.100 volts
   (c) Set $V_X = V_Y = 10$ Vdc and adjust P_3 such that the output voltage is +10.00 volts
   (d) Set $V_X = V_Y = -10$ Vdc. Repeat steps a through d as necessary.

FIGURE 24 — BASIC DIVIDE CIRCUIT

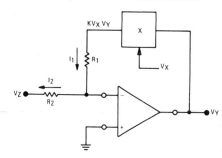

5.3 Divide Circuit

Consider the circuit shown in Figure 24 in which the multiplier is placed in the feedback path of an operational amplifier. For this configuration, the operational amplifier will maintain a "virtual ground" at the inverting (–) input. Assuming that the bias current of the operational amplifier is negligible, then $I_1 = I_2$ and

$$\frac{KV_X V_Y}{R1} = \frac{-V_Z}{R2} \qquad (1)$$

Solving for V_Y,
$$V_Y = \frac{-R1}{R2\,K} \frac{V_Z}{V_X}. \qquad (2)$$

If $R1 = R2$

$$V_Y = \frac{-V_Z}{KV_X} \qquad (3)$$

If $R1 = KR2$

$$V_Y = \frac{-V_Z}{V_X}. \qquad (4)$$

 MOTOROLA *Semiconductor Products Inc.*

OPERATION AND APPLICATIONS INFORMATION (continued)

Hence, the output voltage is the ratio of V_Z to V_X and provides a divide function. This analysis is, of course, the ideal condition. If the multiplier error is taken into account, the output voltage is found to be

$$V_Y = -\left[\frac{R1}{R2\,K}\right]\frac{V_Z}{V_X} + \frac{\triangle E}{K V_X} , \qquad (5)$$

where $\triangle E$ is the error voltage at the output of the multiplier. From this equation, it is seen that divide accuracy is strongly dependent upon the accuracy at which the multiplier can be set, particularly at small values of V_Y. For example, assume that R1 = R2, and K = 1/10. For these conditions the output of the divide circuit is given by:

$$V_Y = \frac{-10\,V_Z}{V_X} + \frac{10\,\triangle E}{V_X} . \qquad (6)$$

From equation 6, it is seen that only when V_X = 10 V is the error voltage of the divide circuit as low as the error of the multiply circuit. For example, when V_X is small, (0.1 volt) the error voltage of the divide circuit can be expected to be a hundred times the error of the basic multiplier circuit.

In terms of percentage error,

$$\text{percentage error} = \frac{\text{error}}{\text{actual}} \times 100\%$$

or from equation (5),

$$P.E._D = \frac{\frac{\triangle E}{K V_X}}{\left[\frac{R1}{R2\,K}\right]\frac{V_Z}{V_X}} = \left[\frac{R2}{R1}\right]\frac{\triangle E}{V_Z} . \qquad (7)$$

From equation 7, the percentage error is inversely related to voltage V_Z (i.e., for increasing values of V_Z, the percentage error decreases).

A circuit that performs the divide function is shown in Figure 25.

Two things should be emphasized concerning Figure 25.
1. The input voltage (V'_X) must be greater than zero and must be positive. This insures that the current out of pin 2 of the multiplier will always be in a direction compatible with the polarity of V_Z.

2. Pins 2 and 14 of the multiplier have been interchanged in respect to the operational amplifiers input terminals. In this instance, Figure 25 differs from the circuit connection shown in Figure 21; necessitated to insure negative feedback around the loop.

A Suggested Adjustment Procedure for the Divide Circuit

1. Set V_Z = 0 volts and adjust the output offset potentiometer (P_4) until the output voltage (V_0) remains at some (not necessarily zero) constant value as V_X' is varied between +1.0 volt and +10 volts.

2. Keep V_Z at 0 volts, set V_X' at +10 volts and adjust the Y input offset potentiometer (P_1) until V_0 = 0 volts.

3. Let $V_X' = V_Z$ and adjust the X input offset potentiometer (P_2) until the output voltage remains at some (not necessarily – 10 volts) constant value as $V_Z = V_X'$ is varied between +1.0 and +10 volts.

4. Keep $V_X' = V_Z$ and adjust the scale factor potentiometer (P_3) until the average value of V_0 is – 10 volts as $V_Z = V_X'$ is varied between +1.0 volt and +10 volts.

5. Repeat steps 1 through 4 as necessary to achieve optimum performance.

5.4 Square Root

A special case of the divide circuit in which the two inputs to the multiplier are connected together is the square root function

FIGURE 25 – DIVIDE CIRCUIT

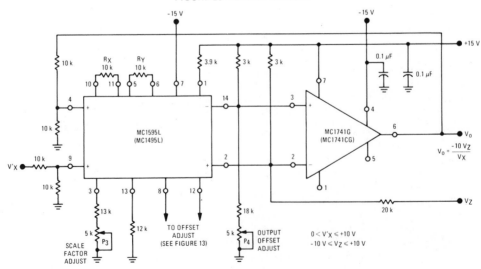

$$V_0 = \frac{-10\,V_Z}{V_X}$$

$0 < V'_X \leqslant +10\,V$
$-10\,V \leqslant V_Z \leqslant +10\,V$

OPERATION AND APPLICATIONS INFORMATION (continued)

FIGURE 26 — BASIC SQUARE ROOT CIRCUIT

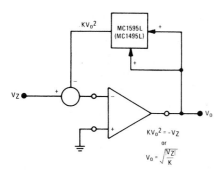

as indicated in Figure 26. This circuit may suffer from latch-up problems similar to those of the divide circuit. Note that only one polarity of input is allowed and diode clamping (see Figure 27) protects against accidental latch-up.

This circuit also may be adjusted in the closed-loop mode as follows:

1. Set V_Z to -0.01 volts and adjust P_4 (output offset) for $V_O = +0.316$ volts, being careful to approach the output from the positive side to preclude the effect of the output diode clamping.

2. Set V_Z to -0.9 volts and adjust P_2 (X adjust) for $V_O = +3.0$ volts.

3. Set V_Z to -10 volts and adjust P_3 (scale factor adjust) for $V_O = +10$ volts.

4. Steps 1 through 3 may be repeated as necessary to achieve desired accuracy.

6. AC Applications

The applications that follow demonstrate the versatility of the monolithic multiplier. If a potted multiplier is used for these cases, the results generally would not be as good because the potted units have circuits that, although they optimize dc multiplication operation, can hinder ac applications.

6.1 Frequency doubling often is done with a diode where the fundamental plus a series of harmonics are generated. However, extensive filtering is required to obtain the desired harmonic, and the second harmonic obtained under this technique usually is small in magnitude and requires amplification.

When a multiplier is used to double frequency the second harmonic is obtained directly, except for a dc term, which can be removed with ac coupling.

$$e_O = KE^2 \cos^2 \omega t$$

$$e_O = \frac{KE^2}{2} (1 + \cos 2\omega t).$$

A potted multiplier can be used to obtain the double frequency component, but frequency would be limited by its internal level-shift amplifier. In the monolithic units, the amplifier is omitted.

In a typical doubler circuit, conventional ± 15-volt supplies are used. An input dynamic range of 5.0 volts peak-to-peak is allowed. The circuit generates wave-forms that are double frequency; less than 1% distortion is encountered without filtering. The configuration has been successfully used in excess of 200 kHz; reducing the scale factor by decreasing the load resistors can further expand the bandwidth.

A slightly modified version of the MC1595 (MC1495) — the MC1596 (MC1496) — has been successfully used as a doubler to obtain 400 MHz. (See Figure 28.)

6.2 Figure 29 represents an application for the monolithic multiplier as a balanced modulator. Here, the audio input signal is 1.6 kHz and the carrier is 40 kHz.

FIGURE 27 — SQUARE ROOT CIRCUIT

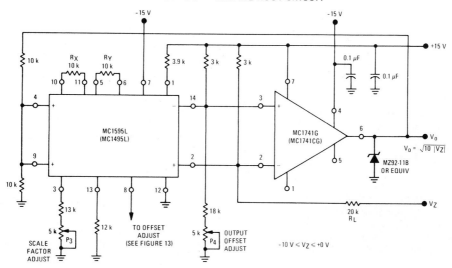

 MOTOROLA *Semiconductor Products Inc.*

OPERATION AND APPLICATIONS INFORMATION (continued)

FIGURE 28 – FREQUENCY DOUBLER

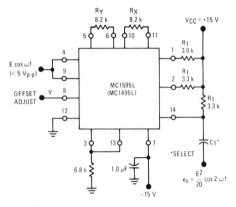

When two equal cosine waves are applied to X and Y, the result is a wave shape of twice the input frequency. For this example the input was a 10 kHz signal, output was 20 kHz.

FIGURE 29 – BALANCED MODULATOR

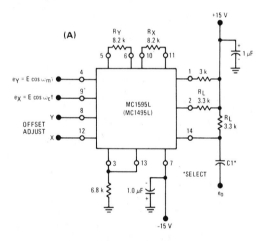

(A)

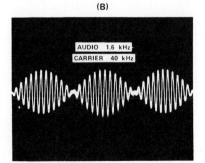

(B)

The defining equation for balanced modulation is

$$K(E_m \cos \omega_m t)(E_c \cos \omega_c t) =$$

$$\frac{KE_c E_m}{2} [\cos(\omega_c + \omega_m)t + \cos(\omega_c - \omega_m)t]$$

where ω_c is the carrier frequency, ω_m is the modulator frequency and K is the multiplier gain constant.

AC coupling at the output eliminates the need for level translation or an operational amplifier; a higher operating frequency results.

A problem common to communications is to extract the intelligence from single-sideband received signal. The ssb signal is of the form

$$e_{ssb} = A \cos(\omega_c + \omega_m)t$$

and if multiplied by the appropriate carrier waveform, $\cos \omega_c t$,

$$e_{ssb} e_{carrier} = \frac{AK}{2} [\cos(2\omega_c + \omega_m)t + \cos(\omega_c)t].$$

If the frequency of the band-limited carrier signal, ω_c, is ascertained in advance the designer can insert a low-pass filter and obtain the $(AK/2) (\cos \omega_c t)$ term with ease. He also can use an operational amplifier for a combination level shift-active filter, as an external component. But in potted multipliers, even if the frequency range can be covered, the operational amplifier is inside and not accessible, so the user must accept the level shifting provided, and still add a low-pass filter.

6.3 Amplitude Modulation

The multiplier performs amplitude modulation, similar to balanced modulation, when a dc term is added to the modulating signal with the Y offset adjust potentiometer. (See Figure 30.)

Here, the identity is

$$E_m(1 + m \cos \omega_m t) E_c \cos \omega_c t = KE_m E_c \cos \omega_c t +$$

$$\frac{KE_m E_c m}{2} [\cos(\omega_c + \omega_m)t + \cos(\omega_c - \omega_m)t]$$

where m indicates the degree of modulation. Since m is adjustable, via potentiometer P_1, 100% modulation is possible. Without extensive tweaking, 96% modulation may be obtained where ω_c and ω_m are the same as in the balanced-modulator example.

6.4 Linear Gain Control

To obtain linear gain control, the designer can feed to one of the two MC1595 (MC1495) inputs a signal that will vary the unit's gain. The following example demonstrates the feasibility of this application. Suppose a 200 kHz sine wave, 1.0 volt peak-to-peak, is the signal to which a gain control will be added. The dynamic range of the control voltage V_C is 0 to +1.0 volt. These must be ascertained and the proper values of R_X and R_Y can be selected for optimum performance. For the 200-kHz operating frequency, load resistors of 100 ohms were chosen to broaden the operating bandwidth of the multiplier, but gain was sacrificed. It may be made up with an amplifier operating at the appropriate frequency. (See Figure 31.)

MOTOROLA *Semiconductor Products Inc.*

OPERATION AND APPLICATIONS INFORMATION (continued)

FIGURE 30 – AMPLITUDE MODULATION

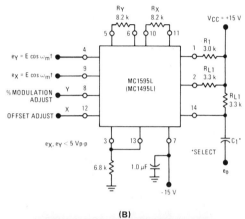

(B)

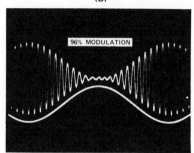

96% MODULATION

The signal is applied to the unit's Y input. Since the total input range is limited to 1.0 volt p-p, a 2.0-volt swing, a current source of 2.0 mA and an R_Y value of 1.0 kilohm is chosen. This takes best advantage of the dynamic range and insures linear operation in the Y-channel.

Since the X input varies between 0 and +1.0 volt, the current source selected was 1.0 mA and the R_X value chosen was 2.0 kilohms. This also insures linear operation over the X input dynamic range.

Choosing R_L = 100 assures wide-bandwidth operation. Hence, the scale factor for this configuration is

$$K = \frac{R_L}{R_X R_Y I_3}$$

$$= \frac{100}{(2\,k)(1\,k)(2 \times 10^{+3})}\,V^{-1}$$

$$= \frac{1}{40}\,V^{-1}.$$

The 2 in the numerator of the equation is missing in this scale-factor expression because the output is single-ended and ac coupled.

To recover the gain, an MC1552 video amplifier with a gain of 40 is used. An operational amplifier also could have been used with frequency compensation to allow a gain of 40 at 200 kHz. The MC1539 operational amplifier can be tailored for this use; and the MC1520 operational amplifier does it directly.

FIGURE 31 – LINEAR GAIN CONTROL

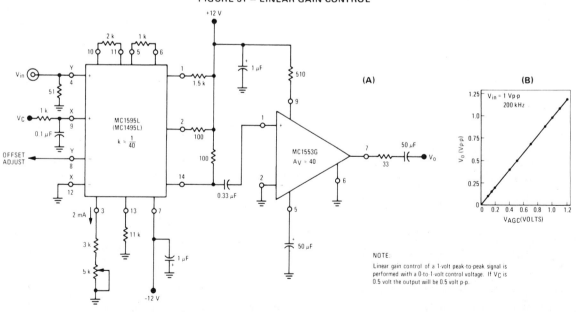

(A)

(B)

NOTE:
Linear gain control of a 1-volt peak-to-peak signal is performed with a 0-to-1-volt control voltage. If V_C is 0.5 volt the output will be 0.5 volt p-p.

Ⓜ **MOTOROLA** *Semiconductor Products Inc.*

OPERATIONS AND APPLICATIONS
INFORMATION INDEX

 MOTOROLA *Semiconductor Products Inc.*

BOX 20912 • PHOENIX ARIZONA 85036 • A SUBSIDIARY OF MOTOROLA INC.

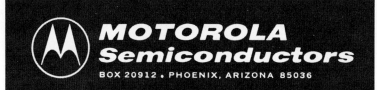

MOTOROLA Semiconductors
BOX 20912 • PHOENIX, ARIZONA 85036

Specifications and Applications Information

QUAD LOW POWER OPERATIONAL AMPLIFIERS

The MC3503 is a low-cost, quad operational amplifier with true differential inputs. The device has electrical characteristics similar to the popular MC1741. However, the MC3503 has several distinct advantages over standard operational amplifier types in single supply applications. The quad amplifier can operate at supply voltages as low as 3.0 Volts or as high as 36 Volts with quiescent currents about one third of those associated with the MC1741 (on a per amplifier basis). The common mode input range includes the negative supply, thereby eliminating the necessity for external biasing components in many applications. The output voltage range also includes the negative power supply voltage.

- Short Circuit Protected Outputs
- Class AB Output Stage for Minimal Crossover Distortion
- True Differential Input Stage
- Single Supply Operation: 3.0 to 36 Volts
- Split Supply Operation: ±1.5 to ±18 Volts
- Low Input Bias Currents: 500 nA Max
- Four Amplifiers Per Package
- Internally Compensated
- Similar Performance to Popular MC1741

QUAD DIFFERENTIAL INPUT OPERATIONAL AMPLIFIERS

SILICON MONOLITHIC INTEGRATED CIRCUIT

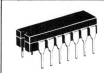

L SUFFIX
CERAMIC PACKAGE
CASE 632
TO-116

P SUFFIX
PLASTIC PACKAGE
CASE 646
(MC3403 and MC3303 only)

SINGLE SUPPLY

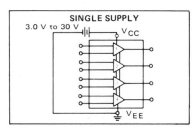

SPLIT SUPPLIES

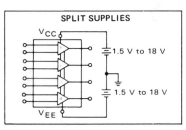

PIN CONNECTIONS

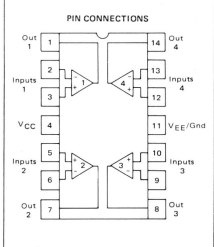

MAXIMUM RATINGS

Rating	Symbol	Value	Unit
Power Supply Voltages			Vdc
Single Supply	V_{CC}	36	
Split Supplies	V_{CC}	+18	
	V_{EE}	−18	
Input Differential Voltage Range (1)	V_{IDR}	±30	Vdc
Input Common Mode Voltage Range (1) (2)	V_{ICR}	±15	Vdc
Storage Temperature Range	T_{stg}		°C
Ceramic Package		−65 to +150	
Plastic Package		−55 to +125	
Operating Ambient Temperature Range	T_A		°C
MC3503		−55 to +125	
MC3403		0 to +70	
MC3303		−40 to +85	
Junction Temperature	T_J		°C
Ceramic Package		175	
Plastic Package		150	

(1) Split Power Supplies.
(2) For Supply Voltages less than ±15 V, the absolute maximum input voltage is equal to the supply voltage.

ORDERING INFORMATION

Type	Temperature Range	Package
MC3303L	−40°C to +85°C	Ceramic DIP
MC3303P	−40°C to +85°C	Plastic DIP
MC3403L	0°C to +70°C	Ceramic DIP
MC3403P	0°C to +70°C	Plastic DIP
MC3503L	−55°C to +125°C	Ceramic DIP

© MOTOROLA INC., 1979　　　　　DS9293 R3

Courtesy of Motorola Inc.

ELECTRICAL CHARACTERISTICS (V$_{CC}$ = +15 V, V$_{EE}$ = –15 V for MC3503, MC3403, V$_{CC}$ = +14 V, V$_{EE}$ = Gnd for MCC3303. T$_A$ = 25°C unless otherwise noted.)

Characteristic	Symbol	MC3503 Min	MC3503 Typ	MC3503 Max	MC3403 Min	MC3403 Typ	MC3403 Max	MC3303 Min	MC3303 Typ	MC3303 Max	Unit
Input Offset Voltage	V$_{IO}$	–	2.0	5.0	–	2.0	10	–	2.0	8.0	mV
T$_A$ = T$_{high}$ to T$_{low}$ (1)		–	–	6.0	–	–	12	–	–	10	
Input Offset Current	I$_{IO}$	–	30	50	–	30	50	–	30	75	nA
T$_A$ = T$_{high}$ to T$_{low}$		–	–	200	–	–	200	–	–	250	
Large Signal Open-Loop Voltage Gain	A$_{VOL}$										V/mV
V$_O$ = ±10 V, R$_L$ = 2.0 kΩ,		50	200	–	20	200	–	20	200	–	
T$_A$ = T$_{high}$ to T$_{low}$		25	300	–	15	–	–	15	–	–	
Input Bias Current	I$_{IB}$	–	–200	–500	–	–200	–500	–	–200	–500	nA
T$_A$ = T$_{high}$ to T$_{low}$		–	–300	–1500	–	–	–800	–	–	–1000	
Output Impedance	z$_o$	–	75	–	–	75	–	–	75	–	Ω
f = 20 Hz											
Input Impedance	z$_i$	0.3	1.0	–	0.3	1.0	–	0.3	1.0	–	MΩ
f = 20 Hz											
Output Voltage Range	V$_{OR}$										V
R$_L$ = 10 kΩ		±12	±13.5	–	±12	±13.5	–	+12	+12.5	–	
R$_L$ = 2.0 kΩ		±10	±13	–	±10	±13	–	+10	+12	–	
R$_L$ = 2.0 kΩ, T$_A$ = T$_{high}$ to T$_{low}$		±10	–	–	±10	–	–	+10	–	–	
Input Common-Mode Voltage Range	V$_{ICR}$	+13 V –V$_{EE}$	+13.5 V –V$_{EE}$	–	+13 V –V$_{EE}$	+13.5 V –V$_{EE}$	–	+13V –V$_{EE}$	+13.5V –V$_{EE}$	–	V
Common-Mode Rejection Ratio	CMRR	70	90	–	70	90	–	70	90	–	dB
R$_S$ ≤ 10 kΩ											
Power Supply Current (V$_O$ = 0)	I$_{CC}$,I$_{EE}$	–	2.8	4.0	–	2.8	7.0	–	2.8	7.0	mA
R$_L$ = ∞											
Individual Output Short-Circuit Current (2)	I$_{OS±}$	±10	±30	±45	±10	±20	±45	±10	±30	±45	mA
Positive Power Supply Rejection Ratio	PSRR+	–	30	150	–	30	150	–	30	150	μV/V
Negative Power Supply Rejection Ratio	PSRR–	–	30	150	–	30	150	–	–	–	μV/V
Average Temperature Coefficient of Input Offset Current	ΔI$_{IO}$/ΔT	–	50	–	–	50	–	–	50	–	pA/°C
T$_A$ = T$_{high}$ to T$_{low}$											
Average Temperature Coefficient of Input Offset Voltage	ΔV$_{IO}$/ΔT	–	10	–	–	10	–	–	10	–	μV/°C
T$_A$ = T$_{high}$ to T$_{low}$											
Power Bandwidth	BW$_p$	–	9.0	–	–	9.0	–	–	9.0	–	kHz
A$_V$ = 1, R$_L$ = 2.0 kΩ, V$_O$ = 20 V(p-p), THD = 5%											
Small-Signal Bandwidth	BW	–	1.0	–	–	1.0	–	–	1.0	–	MHz
A$_V$ = 1, R$_L$ = 10 kΩ, V$_O$ = 50 mV											
Slew Rate	SR	–	0.6	–	–	0.6	–	–	0.6	–	V/μs
A$_V$ = 1, V$_i$ = –10 V to +10 V											
Rise Time	t$_{TLH}$	–	0.35	–	–	0.35	–	–	0.35	–	μs
A$_V$ = 1, R$_L$ = 10 kΩ, V$_O$ = 50 mV											
Fall Time	t$_{THL}$	–	0.35	–	–	0.35	–	–	0.35	–	μs
A$_V$ = 1, R$_L$ = 10 kΩ, V$_O$ = 50 mV											
Overshoot	OS	–	20	–	–	20	–	–	20	–	%
A$_V$ = 1, R$_L$ = 10 kΩ, V$_O$ = 50 mV											
Phase Margin	φm	–	60	–	–	60	–	–	60	–	Degrees
A$_V$ = 1, R$_L$ = 2.0 kΩ, C$_L$ = 200 pF											
Crossover Distortion	–	–	1.0	–	–	1.0	–	–	1.0	–	%
(V$_{in}$ = 30 mVp-p, V$_{out}$ = 2.0 Vp-p, f = 10 kHz)											

(1) T$_{high}$ = 125°C for MC3503, 70°C for MC3403, 85°C for MC3303
  T$_{low}$ = –55°C for MC3503, 0°C for MC3403, –40°C for MC3303

ELECTRICAL CHARACTERISTICS (V$_{CC}$ = 5.0 V, V$_{EE}$ = Gnd, T$_A$ = 25°C unless otherwise noted.)

Characteristic	Symbol	MC3503 Min	MC3503 Typ	MC3503 Max	MC3403 Min	MC3403 Typ	MC3403 Max	MC3303 Min	MC3303 Typ	MC3303 Max	Unit
Input Offset Voltage	V$_{IO}$	–	2.0	5.0	–	2.0	10	–	–	10	mV
Input Offset Current	I$_{IO}$	–	30	50	–	30	50	–	–	75	nA
Input Bias Current	I$_{IB}$	–	–200	–500	–	–200	–500	–	–	–500	nA
Large-Signal Open-Loop Voltage Gain	A$_{VOL}$	10	200	–	10	200	–	10	200	–	V/mV
R$_L$ = 2.0 kΩ											
Power Supply Rejection Ratio	PSRR	–	–	150	–	–	150	–	–	150	μV/V
Output Voltage Range (3)	V$_{OR}$										Vp-p
R$_L$ = 10 kΩ, V$_{CC}$ = 5.0 V		3.3	3.5	–	3.3	3.5	–	3.3	3.5	–	
R$_L$ = 10 kΩ, 5.0 V ≤ V$_{CC}$ ≤ 30 V		V$_{CC}$–1.7	V$_{CC}$–1.5	–	V$_{CC}$–1.7	V$_{CC}$–1.5	–	V$_{CC}$–1.7	V$_{CC}$–1.5	–	
Power Supply Current	I$_{CC}$	–	2.5	4.0	–	2.5	7.0	–	2.5	7.0	mA
Channel Separation	–	–	–120	–	–	–120	–	–	–120	–	dB
f = 1.0 kHz to 20 kHz (Input Referenced)											

(2) Not to exceed maximum package power dissipation.
(3) Output will swing to ground

 MOTOROLA *Semiconductor Products Inc.*

CIRCUIT SCHEMATIC

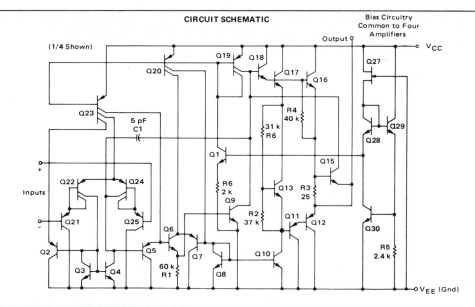

(1/4 Shown)

Bias Circuitry
Common to Four
Amplifiers

INVERTER PULSE RESPONSE

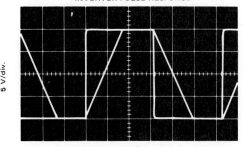

5 V/div.

20 µs/div.

CIRCUIT DESCRIPTION

The MC3503/3403/3303 is made using four internally compensated, two-stage operational amplifiers. The first stage of each consists of differential input devices Q24 and Q22 with input buffer transistors Q25 and Q21 and the differential to single ended converter Q3 and Q4. The first stage performs not only the first stage gain function but also performs the level shifting and transconductance reduction functions. By reducing the transconductance a smaller compensation capacitor (only 5 pF) can be employed, thus saving chip area. The transconductance reduction is accomplished by splitting the collectors of Q24 and Q22. Another feature of this input stage is that the input common-mode range can include the negative supply or ground, in single supply operation,

without saturating either the input devices or the differential to single-ended converter. The second stage consists of a standard current source load amplifier stage.

The output stage is unique because it allows the output to swing to ground in single supply operation and yet does not exhibit any crossover distortion in split supply operation. This is possible because class AB operation is utilized.

Each amplifier is biased from an internal-voltage regulator which has a low temperature coefficient thus giving each amplifier good temperature characteristics as well as excellent power supply rejection.

THERMAL INFORMATION

The maximum power consumption an integrated circuit can tolerate at a given operating ambient temperature, can be found from the equation:

$$P_{D(T_A)} = \frac{T_{J(max)} - T_A}{R_{\theta JA}(Typ)}$$

Where: $P_{D(T_A)}$ = Power Dissipation allowable at a given operating ambient temperature. This must be greater than the sum of the products of the supply voltages and supply currents at the worst case operating condition.

$T_{J(max)}$ = Maximum Operating Junction Temperature as listed in the Maximum Ratings Section

T_A = Maximum Desired Operating Ambient Temperature

$R_{\theta JA}(Typ)$ = Typical Thermal Resistance Junction to Ambient

OUTLINE DIMENSIONS

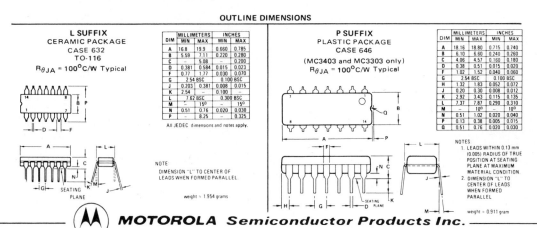

L SUFFIX
CERAMIC PACKAGE
CASE 632
TO-116
$R_{\theta JA}$ = 100°C/W Typical

DIM	MILLIMETERS MIN	MAX	INCHES MIN	MAX
A	16.8	19.9	0.660	0.785
B	5.59	7.11	0.220	0.280
C	–	5.08	–	0.200
D	0.381	0.584	0.015	0.023
F	0.77	1.77	0.030	0.070
G	2.54 BSC		0.100 BSC	
J	0.203	0.381	0.008	0.015
K	2.54		0.100	
L	7.62 BSC		0.300 BSC	
M		15°		15°
N	0.51	0.76	0.020	0.030
P	–	8.25	–	0.325

All JEDEC dimensions and notes apply.

NOTE:
DIMENSION "L" TO CENTER OF LEADS WHEN FORMED PARALLEL.

weight = 1.954 grams

P SUFFIX
PLASTIC PACKAGE
CASE 646

(MC3403 and MC3303 only)
$R_{\theta JA}$ = 100°C/W Typical

DIM	MILLIMETERS MIN	MAX	INCHES MIN	MAX
A	18.16	18.80	0.715	0.740
B	6.10	6.60	0.240	0.260
C	4.06	4.57	0.160	0.180
D	0.38	0.51	0.015	0.020
F	1.02	1.52	0.040	0.060
G	2.54 BSC		0.100 BSC	
J	1.32	1.83	0.052	0.072
J	0.20	0.30	0.008	0.012
K	2.92	3.43	0.115	0.135
L	7.37	7.87	0.290	0.310
M	–	10°	–	10°
N	0.51	1.02	0.020	0.040
P	0.13	0.38	0.005	0.015
Q	0.51	0.76	0.020	0.030

NOTES:
1. LEADS WITHIN 0.13 mm (0.005) RADIUS OF TRUE POSITION AT SEATING PLANE AT MAXIMUM MATERIAL CONDITION.
2. DIMENSION "L" TO CENTER OF LEADS WHEN FORMED PARALLEL.

weight = 0.911 gram

MOTOROLA *Semiconductor Products Inc.*

TYPICAL PERFORMANCE CURVES

FIGURE 1 — SINE WAVE RESPONSE

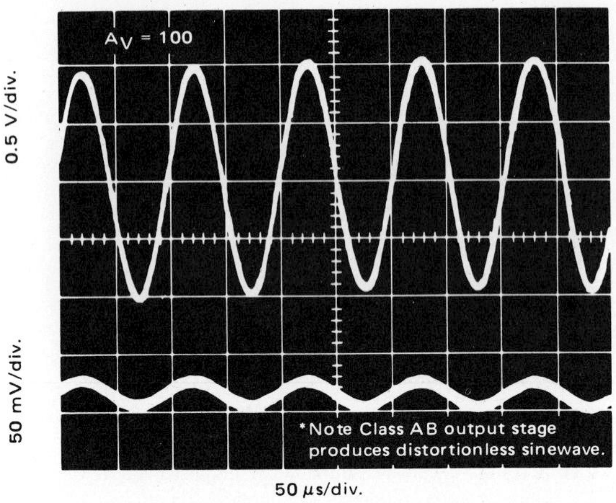

$A_V = 100$

0.5 V/div.

50 mV/div.

*Note Class AB output stage produces distortionless sinewave.

50 μs/div.

FIGURE 2 — OPEN LOOP FREQUENCY RESPONSE

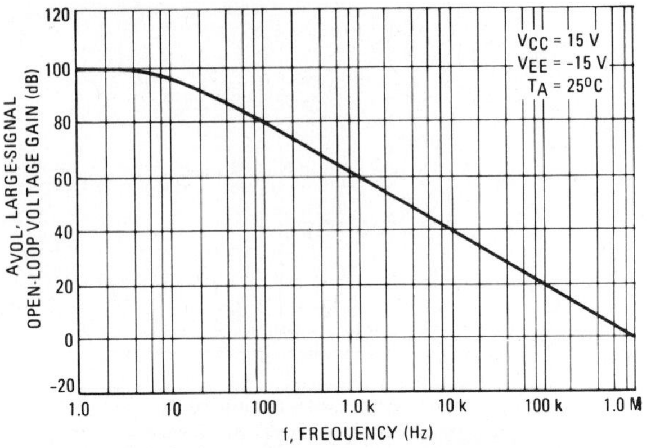

$V_{CC} = 15$ V
$V_{EE} = -15$ V
$T_A = 25°C$

A_{VOL}, LARGE-SIGNAL OPEN-LOOP VOLTAGE GAIN (dB)

f, FREQUENCY (Hz)

FIGURE 3 — POWER BANDWIDTH

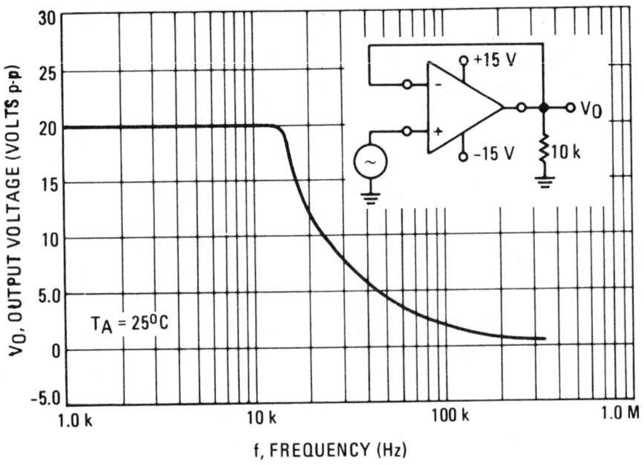

V_O, OUTPUT VOLTAGE (VOLTS p-p)

$T_A = 25°C$

+15 V
−15 V
V_O
10 k

f, FREQUENCY (Hz)

FIGURE 4 — OUTPUT SWING versus SUPPLY VOLTAGE

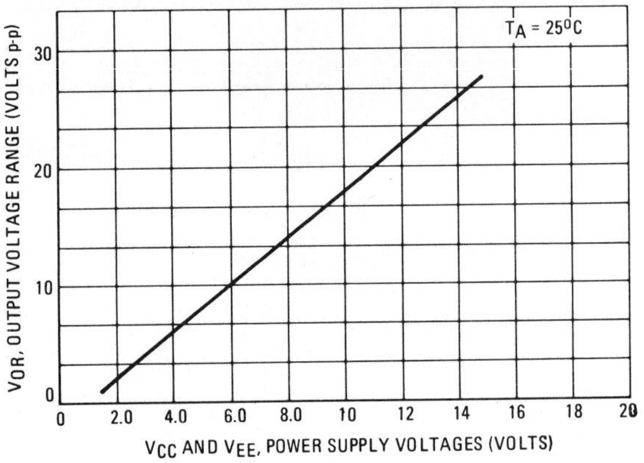

$T_A = 25°C$

V_{OR}, OUTPUT VOLTAGE RANGE (VOLTS p-p)

V_{CC} AND V_{EE}, POWER SUPPLY VOLTAGES (VOLTS)

FIGURE 5 — INPUT BIAS CURRENT versus TEMPERATURE

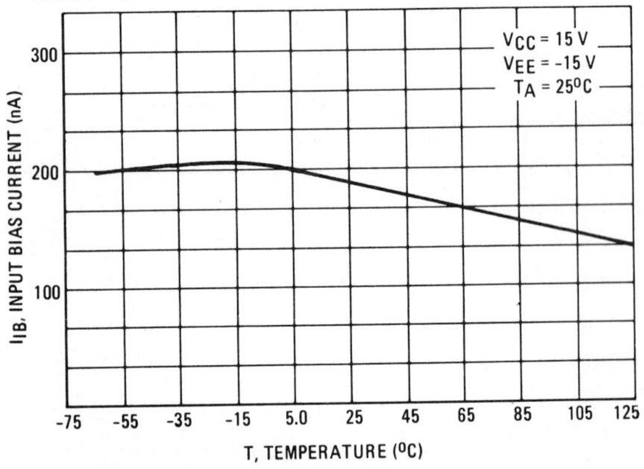

$V_{CC} = 15$ V
$V_{EE} = -15$ V
$T_A = 25°C$

I_{IB}, INPUT BIAS CURRENT (nA)

T, TEMPERATURE (°C)

FIGURE 6 — INPUT BIAS CURRENT versus SUPPLY VOLTAGE

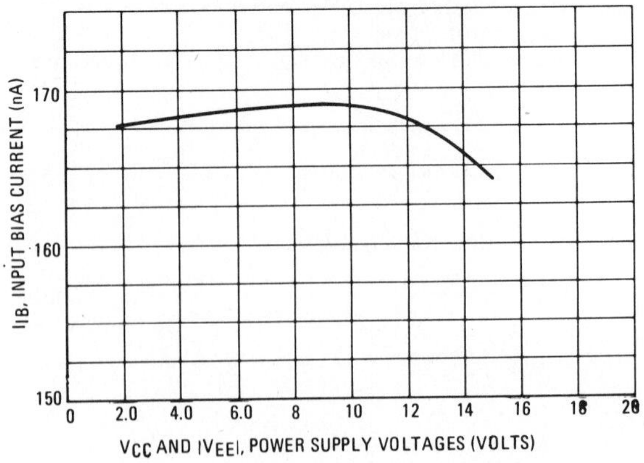

I_{IB}, INPUT BIAS CURRENT (nA)

V_{CC} AND $|V_{EE}|$, POWER SUPPLY VOLTAGES (VOLTS)

MOTOROLA *Semiconductor Products Inc.*

National Semiconductor

Operational Amplifiers/Buffers

LM1900/LM2900/LM3900, LM3301, LM3401 quad amplifiers

general description

The LM1900 series consists of four independent, dual input, internally compensated amplifiers which were designed specifically to operate off of a single power supply voltage and to provide a large output voltage swing. These amplifiers make use of a current mirror to achieve the non-inverting input function. Application areas include: ac amplifiers, RC active filters, low frequency triangle, squarewave and pulse waveform generation circuits, tachometers and low speed, high voltage digital logic gates.

features

- Wide single supply voltage 4 V$_{DC}$ to 36 V$_{DC}$
  range or dual supplies ±2 V$_{DC}$ to ±18 V$_{DC}$
- Supply current drain independent of supply voltage
- Low input biasing current 30 nA
- High open-loop gain 70 dB
- Wide bandwidth 2.5 MHz (Unity Gain)
- Large output voltage swing (V$^+$ −1) Vp-p
- Internally frequency compensated for unity gain
- Output short-circuit protection

schematic and connection diagrams

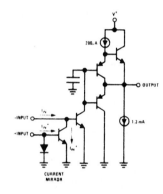

Order Number LM1900D
or LM2900D
See NS Package D14E
Order Number LM1900J
or LM2900J
See NS Package J14A
Order Number LM2900N,
LM3900N, LM3301N
or LM3401N
See NS Package N14A

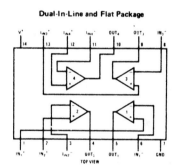

Dual-In-Line and Flat Package

typical applications (V$^+$ = 15 V$_{DC}$)

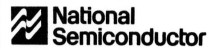

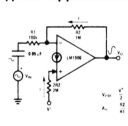

Inverting Amplifier

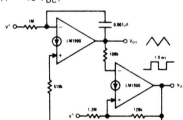

Triangle/Square Generator

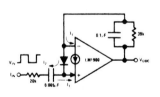

Frequency-Doubling Tachometer

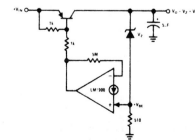

Low V$_{IN}$ − V$_{OUT}$ Voltage Regulator

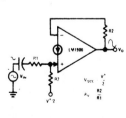

Non-Inverting Amplifier

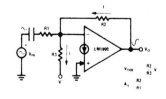

Negative Supply Biasing

Courtesy of National Semiconductor Corporation

absolute maximum ratings

	LM1900	LM2900/LM3900	LM3301	LM3401
Supply Voltage	36 VDC / ±18 VDC	32 VDC / ±16 VDC	28 VDC / ±14 VDC	18 VDC / ±9 VDC
Power Dissipation (T_A = 25°C) (Note 1)				
Cavity DIP	900 mW	900 mW		
Flat Pack	800 mW	800 mW		
Molded DIP	570 mW	570 mW	570 mW	570 mW
Input Currents, I_{IN}^+ or I_{IN}	20 mADC	20 mADC	20 mADC	20 mADC
Output Short-Circuit Duration — One Amplifier T_A = 25°C (See Application Hints)	Continuous	Continuous	Continuous	Continuous
Operating Temperature Range	−55°C to +125°C	LM2900 −40°C to +85°C LM3900 0°C to +70°C	−40°C to +85°C	0°C to +75°C
Storage Temperature Range	−65°C to +150°C	−65°C to +150°C	−65°C to +150°C	−65°C to +150°C
Lead Temperature (Soldering, 10 seconds)	300°C	300°C	300°C	300°C

electrical characteristics (Note 6)

PARAMETER	CONDITIONS	LM1900 MIN	TYP	MAX	LM2900 MIN	TYP	MAX	LM3900 MIN	TYP	MAX	LM3301 MIN	TYP	MAX	LM3401 MIN	TYP	MAX	UNITS
Open Loop																	
Voltage Gain	T_A = 25°C, f = 100 Hz	2	3											800			V/mV
Voltage Gain	T_A = 25°C, Inverting Input				1.2	2.8		1.2	2.8		1.2	2.8		1.2	2.8		V/mV
Input Resistance			1			1			1			1		0.1	1		MΩ
Output Resistance			8			8			8			8			8		kΩ
Unity Gain Bandwidth	T_A = 25°C, Inverting Input		2.5			2.5			2.5			2.5			2.5		MHz
Input Bias Current	T_A = 25°C, Inverting Input		25	100		30	200		30	200		30	300		30	300	nA
	Inverting Input															500	nA
Slew Rate	T_A = 25°C, Positive Output Swing		0.5			0.5			0.5			0.5			0.5		V/µs
	T_A = 25°C, Negative Output Swing		20			20			20			20			20		V/µs
Supply Current	T_A = 25°C, R_L = ∞ On All Amplifiers		6.2	12		6.2	10		6.2	10		6.2	10		6.2	10	mADC
Output Voltage Swing	T_A = 25°C, R_L = 2k, V_{CC} = 15.0 V_{DC}																
V_{OUT} High	I_{IN} = 0, I_{IN}^+ = 0	13.5	14.2		13.5			13.5			13.5			13.5			VDC
V_{OUT} Low	I_{IN} = 10µA, I_{IN}^+ = 0		0.09	0.2		0.09	0.2		0.09	0.2		0.09	0.2		0.09	0.2	VDC
V_{OUT} High	I_{IN} = 0, I_{IN}^+ = 0 R_L = ∞, V_{CC} = 30 V_{DC}	28.0	29.5			29.5			29.5			29.5			29.5		VDC
Output Current Capability	T_A = 25°C																
Source	(Note 2)	10	15		6	18		6	10		5	18		5	10		mADC
Sink	(Note 2)	1.0	1.3		0.5	1.3		0.5	1.3		0.5	1.3		0.5	1.3		mADC
I_{SINK}	V_{OL} = 1V, I_{IN} = 5µA	4	5			5			5			5			5		mADC

electrical characteristics (con't) (Note 6)

PARAMETER	CONDITIONS	LM1900			LM2900			LM3900			LM3301			LM3401			UNITS
		MIN	TYP	MAX	MIN	TYP	MAX	MIN	TYP	MAX	MIN	TYP	MAX	MIN	TYP	MAX	
Power Supply Rejection	$T_A = 25°C$, f = 100 Hz	50	70			70			70			70			70		dB
Mirror Gain	@ 20µA (Note 3)	0.95	1.0	1.05	0.90	1.0	1.1	0.90	1.0	1.1	0.90	1	1.10	0.90	1	1.10	µA/µA
	@ 200µA (Note 3)	0.95	1.0	1.05	0.90	1.0	1.1	0.90	1.0	1.1	0.90	1	1.10	0.90	1	1.10	µA/µA
ΔMirror Gain	@ 20µA To 200µA (Note 3)		1	2		2	5		2	5		2	5		2	5	%
Mirror Current	(Note 4)		10	500		10	500		10	500		10	500		10	500	µADC
Negative Input Current	$T_A = 25°C$ (Note 5)		1.0			1.0			1.0			1.0			1.0		mADC
Voltage Gain	f = 100 Hz	800															V/mV
Input Bias Current	Inverting Input			150													nA

Note 1: For operating at high temperatures, the device must be derated based on a 125°C maximum junction temperature and a thermal resistance of 175°C/W which applies for the device soldered in a printed circuit board, operating in a still air ambient.

Note 2: The output current sink capability can be increased for large signal conditions by overdriving the inverting input. This is shown in the section on Typical Characteristics.

Note 3: This spec indicates the current gain of the current mirror which is used as the non-inverting input.

Note 4: Input V_{BE} match between the non-inverting and the inverting inputs occurs for a mirror current (non-inverting input current) of approximately 10µA. This is therefore a typical design center for many of the application circuits.

Note 5: Clamp transistors are included on the IC to prevent the input voltages from swinging below ground more than approximately $-0.3~V_{DS}$. The negative input currents which may result from large signal overdrive with capacitance input coupling need to be externally limited to values of approximately 1 mA. Negative input currents in excess of 4 mA will cause the output voltage to drop to a low voltage. This maximum current applies to any one of the input terminals. If more than one of the input terminals are simultaneously driven negative smaller maximum currents are allowed. Common-mode current biasing can be used to prevent negative input voltages; see for example, the "Differentiator Circuit" in the applications section.

Note 6: These specs apply for $-55°C \leq T_A \leq +125°C$, unless otherwise stated.

typical performance characteristics

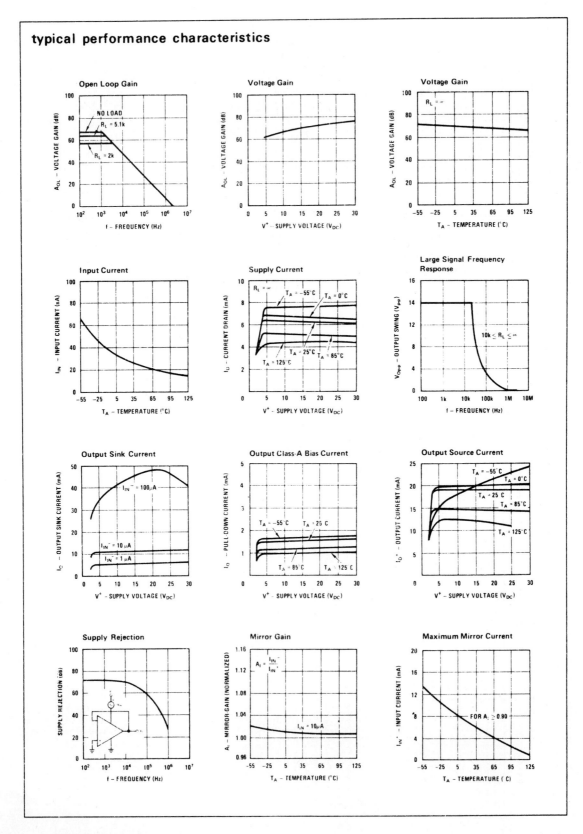

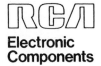

Electronic Components

CA3050
CA3051

Dual Differential Amplifiers
Monolithic Silicon

The CA3050 and CA3051 each consists of two differential amplifiers with associated constant current transistors on a common substrate. Each amplifier is driven by Darlington-connected emitter follower inputs to provide high input impedance, low bias current, and low offset current. A string of diodes is included to provide temperature-compensated bias to the constant current transistors and a low impedance bias point for the inputs to the differential amplifiers when a single power supply is used.

The CA3050 is supplied in an hermetic 14-lead Dual-In-Line ceramic package rated for operation over the full military temperature range of -55°C to +125°C.

The CA3051 is supplied in a Dual-In-Line plastic package for applications requiring only a limited temperature range of -25°C to +85°C.

TWO DARLINGTON-CONNECTED DIFFERENTIAL AMPLIFIERS WITH DIODE BIAS STRING

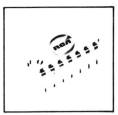

CA3050

For Low-Power Applications at Frequencies from DC to 20 MHz

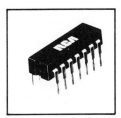

CA3051

FEATURES
- Input offset current .... 70 nA max.
- Input bias current .... 500 nA max.
- Input offset voltage .... 5 mV max.
- Input impedance .... 460 kΩ typ.
- Independently accessible inputs and outputs

APPLICATIONS
- Matched dual amplifiers
- Dual sense amplifiers
- Dual Schmitt triggers
- Dual multivibrators
- Doubly balanced detectors and modulators
- Balanced quadrature detectors
- Synthesizer mixers
- Product detectors

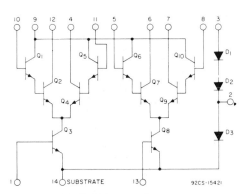

Fig.1 - Schematic diagram.

Courtesy of RCA

Printed in U.S.A./3-70

Reprinted from Issue dated 11-68

ELECTRICAL CHARACTERISTICS at T_A = 25°C

CHARACTERISTICS	SYMBOLS	TEST CONDITIONS	TEST CIRCUIT FIG.	LIMITS CA3050/CA3051			UNITS	TYPICAL CHARACTERISTICS CURVES FIG.
				MIN.	TYP.	MAX.		
STATIC								
Amplifier Characteristics								
Input Offset Voltage	V_{IO}	V_{CC} = 6 V, I_3 = 2 mA	–	–	1.5	5	mV	2a,b
Input Offset Current	I_{IO}	V_{CC} = 6 V, I_3 = 2 mA	–	–	7	70	nA	3a,b
Input Bias Current	I_I	V_{CC} = 6 V, I_3 = 2 mA	–	–	200	500	nA	4a,b
Quiescent Operating Current Ratio	$\left\|\dfrac{(I_4+I_{12})\ \text{or}\ (I_6+I_7)}{I_3}\right\|$	V_{CC} = 6 V, I_3 = 2 mA	–	0.9	1.00	1.13	–	5a,b
DC Forward Base-to-Emitter Voltage	V_{BE}	V_{CE} = 3 V $\begin{cases} I_C = 50\,\mu A \\ 1\ mA \\ 3\ mA \\ 10\ mA \end{cases}$	– – – –	– – – –	0.645 0.725 0.760 0.805	0.700 0.800 0.850 0.900	V	6
Temperature Coefficient of Base-to-Emitter Voltage	$\dfrac{\triangle V_{BE}}{\triangle T}$	V_{CE} = 3 V, I_C = 1 mA	–	–	-1.9	–	mV/°C	7
Transistor Characteristics								
Collector-Cutoff Current	I_{CBO}	V_{CB} = 10 V, I_E = 0	–	–	0.002	100	nA	8
Collector-to-Emitter Breakdown Voltage	$V_{(BR)CEO}$	I_C = 1 mA, I_B = 0	–	15	24	–	V	–
Collector-to-Base Breakdown Voltage	$V_{(BR)CBO}$	I_C = 10 μA, I_E = 0	–	20	60	–	V	–
Collector-to-Substrate Breakdown Voltage	$V_{(BR)CIO}$	I_C = 10 μA, I_{CI} = 0	–	20	60	–	V	–
Emitter-to-Base Breakdown Voltage	$V_{(BR)EBO}$	I_E = 10 μA, I_C = 0	–	5	7	–	V	–
DYNAMIC								
Transistor Characteristics								
Emitter-to-Base Capacitance	C_{EB}	V_{EB} = 3 V, I_E = 0	–	–	0.78	–	pF	9
Collector-to-Base Capacitance	C_{CB}	V_{CB} = 3 V, I_C = 0	–	–	0.47	–	pF	9
Collector-to-Substrate Capacitance	C_{CI}	V_{CS} = 3 V, I_C = 0	–	–	1.92	–	pF	9
Amplifier Characteristics								
Gain-Bandwidth Product (For Single Transistor)	f_T	V_{CE} = 5 V, I_C = 3 mA	–	–	600	--	MHz	10
Forward Transadmittance (With single-ended input and output)	$\|y_{21}\|$	V_{CC} = 10 V, I_3 = 2 mA, f = 1 MHz	11	7	9	11	mmho	11
Bandwidth at -3 dB Point	BW	V_{CC} = 10 V, I_3 = 2 mA	11	–	4.3	–	MHz	11
Input Impedance	Z_{IN}	V_{CC} = 10 V, I_3 = 2 mA, f = 1 KHz	12	–	460	–	kΩ	12
Output Impedance	Z_{OUT}	I_3 = 2 mA, f = 1 KHz	13	–	170	–	kΩ	13
Common-Mode Rejection Ratio	CMR	I_3 = 2 mA, f = 1 KHz	–	–	65	–	dB	–
AGC Range	AGC	I_3 = 2 mA, f = 1 KHz, Terminal No.3 Grounded	11	–	60	–	dB	–

MAXIMUM RATINGS, ABSOLUTE-MAXIMUM VALUES, AT $T_A = 25°C$

	CA3050	CA3051	
Power Dissipation, P:			
Any one transistor	150	150	mW
Total package	900	750	mW
For $T_A > 55°C$, Derate at . .	8	6.67	mW/°C
Temperature Range:			
Operating	-55 to +125	-25 to +85	°C
Storage	-65 to +200	-25 to +85	°C

The following ratings apply for each transistor in the device:

Collector-to-Emitter Voltage, V_{CEO}	15	V
Collector-to-Base Voltage, V_{CBO}	20	V
Collector-to-Substrate Voltage, V_{CIO}*	20	V
Emitter-to-Base Voltage, V_{EBO}	5	V
Collector Current, I_C	50	mA

* The collector of each transistor of the CA3050 and CA3051 is isolated from the substrate by an integral diode. *The substrate (terminal 14) must be more negative than all col-* lectors *to maintain isolation between transistors and to provide for normal transistor action.*

MAXIMUM VOLTAGE RATINGS

The following chart gives the range of voltages which can be applied to the terminals listed vertically with respect to the terminals listed horizontally. For example, the voltage range between vertical terminal 2 and horizontal terminal 3 is +5 to -2 volts.

TERM-INAL No.	1	2	3	4	5	6	7	8	9	10	11	12	13	14
1	–	*	*	*	*	*	*	*	*	*	*	*	*	+1 -5
2			+5 -2	*	*	*	*	*	*	*	*	*	*	+1 -1
3				*	*	*	*	*	*	*	*	*	*	+3 -1
4					*	*	*	*	*	+14 -2.5 Note 3	+14 -2.5 Note 4	*	*	+20 -1
5						+2.5 -14 Note 1	+2.5 -14 Note 1	+10 -10	+1 -20	*	*	*	*	+16 -
6							*	+14 -2.5 Note 2	*	*	*	*	*	+20 -1
7								+14 -2.5 Note 2	*	*	*	*	*	+20 -1
8									+1 -20	*	*	*	*	+16 -
9										+20 -1	+20 -1	*	*	+20 -1
10											+10 -10	+2.5 -14 Note 3	*	+16 -
11												+2.5 -14 Note 4	*	+16 -
12														+20 -1
13														+1 -5
14														Ref. Substrate

MAXIMUM CURRENT RATINGS

TERM-INAL No.	I_{IN} mA	I_{OUT} mA
1	5	0 1
2	50	50
3	50	1
4	50	1
5	5	0 1
6	50	1
7	50	1
8	5	0 1
9	50	1
10	5	0 1
11	5	0.1
12	50	1
13	5	0 1
14	100	5

Note 1: This rating is important only when terminal 5 is more positive than terminal 8.

Note 2: This rating is important only when terminal 8 is more positive than terminal 5.

Note 3: This rating is important only when terminal 10 is more positive than terminal 11.

Note 4: This rating is important only when terminal 11 is more positive than terminal 10.

* Voltages are not normally applied between these terminals. Voltages appearing between these terminals will be safe if the specified limits between all other terminals are not exceeded.

TYPICAL STATIC CHARACTERISTICS

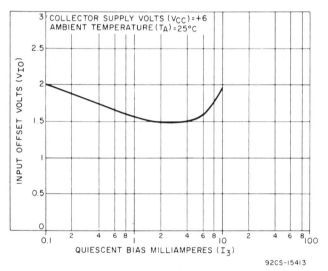

Fig.2(a) - Typical input offset voltage vs quiescent bias current.

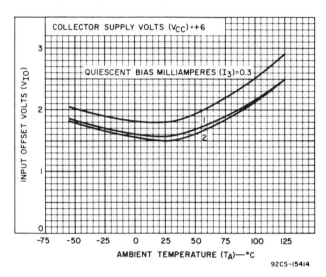

Fig.2(b) - Typical input offset voltage vs ambient temperature.

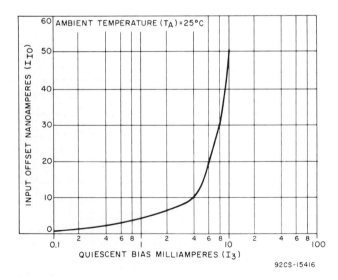

Fig.3(a) - Typical input offset current vs quiescent bias current.

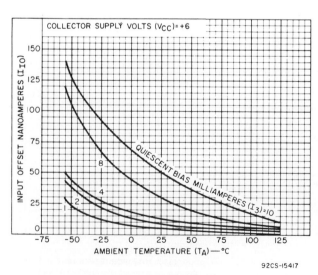

Fig.3(b) - Typical input offset current vs ambient temperature.

STATIC CHARACTERISTICS

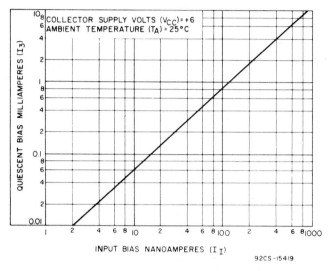

Fig.4(a) - Typical quiescent bias current vs input bias current.

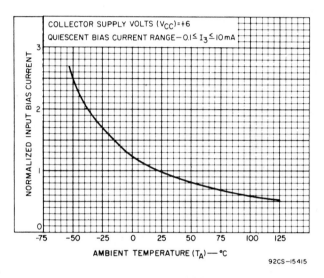

Fig.4(b) - Typical normalized input bias current vs ambient temperature.

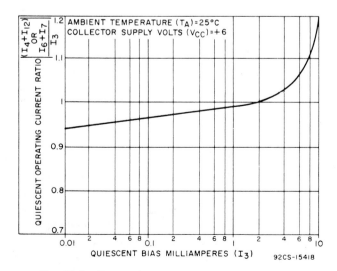

Fig.5(a) - Typical quiescent operating current ratio vs quiescent bias current.

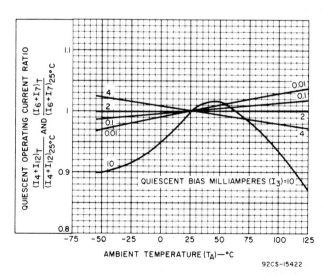

Fig.5(b) - Typical quiescent operating current ratio vs ambient temperature.

STATIC CHARACTERISTICS

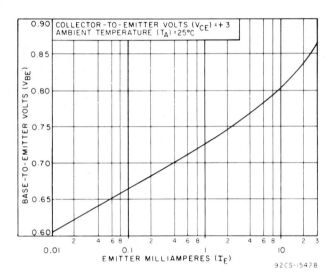

Fig.6 - *Typical static base-to-emitter voltage characteristic vs emitter current for all transistors and forward diode voltage drops.*

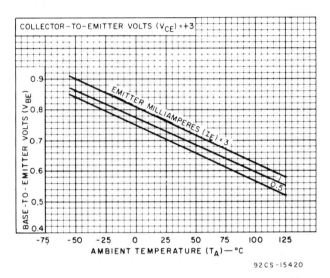

Fig.7 - *Typical base-to-emitter voltage characteristic vs ambient temperature for each transistor.*

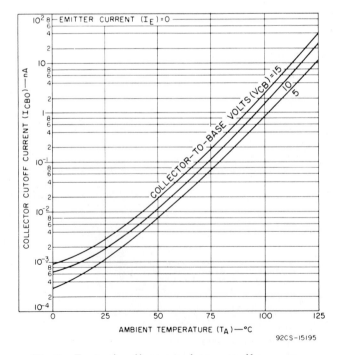

Fig.8 - *Typical collector-to-base cutoff current vs ambient temperature for each transistor.*

DYNAMIC CHARACTERISTICS FOR EACH TRANSISTOR

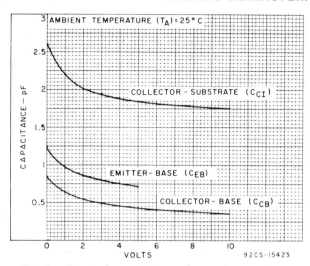

Fig.9 - *Typical capacitance for each transistor.*

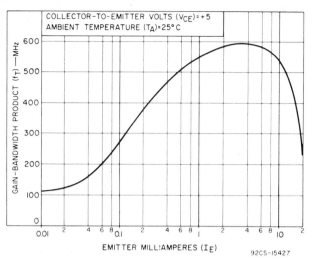

Fig.10 - *Typical gain-bandwidth product (f_T) for each transistor vs emitter current.*

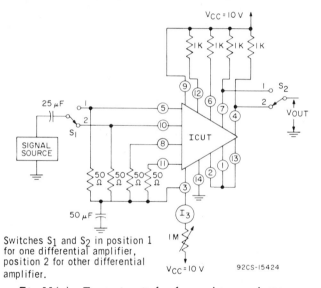

Switches S_1 and S_2 in position 1 for one differential amplifier, position 2 for other differential amplifier.

Fig.11(a) - *Test circuit for forward transadmittance, -3 dB bandwidth, and AGC range.*

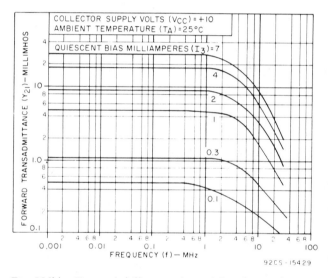

Fig.11(b) - *Typical differential amplifier forward transadmittance with single-ended output vs frequency.*

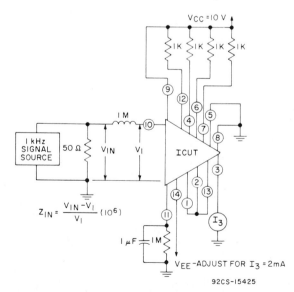

Fig.12(a) - *Test circuit for input impedance.*

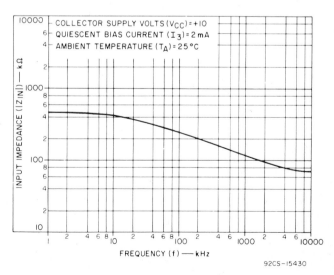

Fig.12(b) - *Typical input impedance vs frequency with output short-circuited.*

DYNAMIC CHARACTERISTICS FOR EACH TRANSISTOR

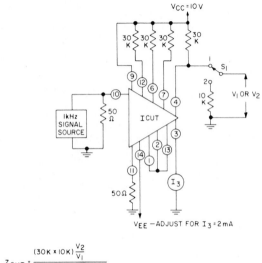

$$Z_{OUT} = \frac{(30K \times 10K)\frac{V_2}{V_1}}{\frac{V_2}{V_1}(30K + 10K) - 10K}$$

92CS-15426

Fig.13(a) - Test circuit for output impedance.

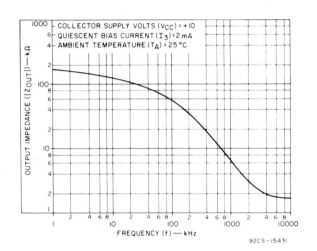

92CS-15431

Fig.13(b) - Typical output impedance vs frequency with input short-circuited.

DIMENSIONAL OUTLINE CA3050

14-Lead Dual In-Line
Ceramic Package JEDEC TO-116

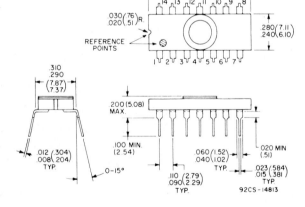

DIMENSIONAL OUTLINE CA3051

14-Lead Dual In-Line
Plastic Package JEDEC TO-116

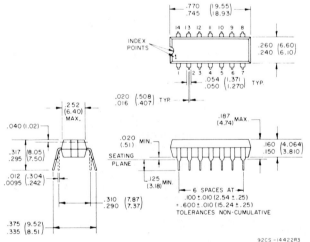

92CS-14422R3

RCA | Electronic Components | Harrison, N.J. 07029

TYPES TL070, TL070A, TL071, TL071A, TL071B, TL072, TL072A, TL072B, TL074, TL074A, TL074B, TL075
LOW-NOISE JFET-INPUT OPERATIONAL AMPLIFIERS

BULLETIN NO. DL-S 12640, SEPTEMBER 1978

20 DEVICES COVER COMMERCIAL, INDUSTRIAL, AND MILITARY TEMPERATURE RANGES

- Low Noise . . . V_n = 18 nV/$\sqrt{Hz}$ Typ

- Low Harmonic Distortion . . . 0.01% Typ

- Wide Common-Mode and Differential Voltage Ranges

- Low Input Bias and Offset Currents

- Output Short-Circuit Protection

- High Input Impedance . . . JFET-Input Stage

- Internal Frequency Compensation

- Low Power Consumption

- Latch-Up-Free Operation

- High Slew Rate . . . 13 V/μs Typ

description

The JFET-input operational amplifiers of the TL071 series are designed as low-noise versions of the TL081 series amplifiers with low input bias and offset currents and fast slew rate. The low harmonic distortion and low noise make the TL071 series ideally suited as amplifiers for high-fidelity and audio preamplifier applications. Each amplifier features JFET-inputs (for high input impedance) coupled with bipolar output stages all integrated on a single monolithic chip.

Device types with an "M" suffix are characterized for operation over the full military temperature range of −55°C to 125°C, those with an "I" suffix are characterized for operation from −25°C to 85°C, and those with a "C" suffix are characterized for operation from 0°C to 70°C.

TL070, TL070A

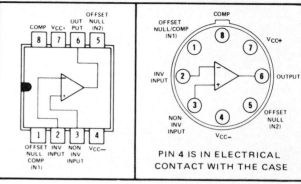

TL071, TL071A, TL071B

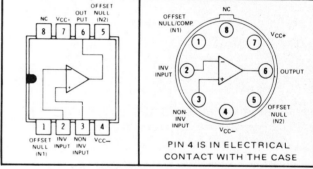

TL072, TL072A, TL072B

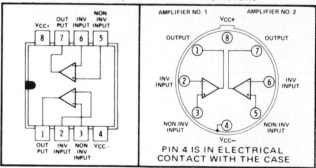

TL074, TL074A, TL074B
J OR N DUAL-IN-LINE PACKAGE (TOP VIEW)

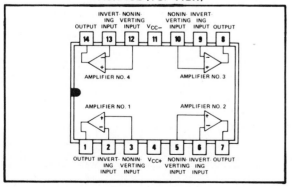

TL075
N DUAL-IN-LINE PACKAGE (TOP VIEW)

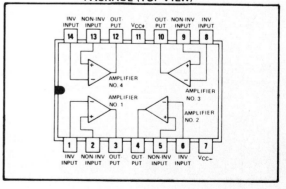

schematic (each amplifier)

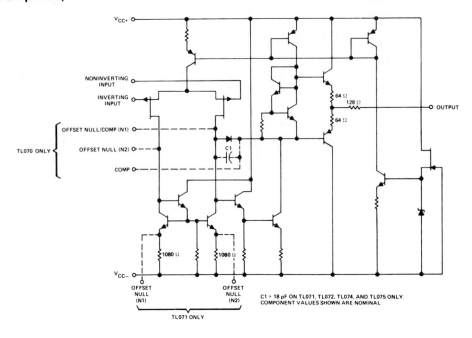

C1 ≈ 18 pF ON TL071, TL072, TL074, AND TL075 ONLY.
COMPONENT VALUES SHOWN ARE NOMINAL

absolute maximum ratings over operating free-air temperature range (unless otherwise noted)

		TL07_M	TL07_I	TL07_C TL07_AC TL07_BC	UNIT
Supply voltage, $V_{CC}+$ (see Note 1)		18	18	18	V
Supply voltage, $V_{CC}-$ (see Note 1)		−18	−18	−18	V
Differential input voltage (see Note 2)		±30	±30	±30	V
Input voltage (see Notes 1 and 3)		±15	±15	±15	V
Duration of output short circuit (see Note 4)		Unlimited	Unlimited	Unlimited	
Continuous total dissipation at (or below) 25°C free-air	J, JG, N, or P Package	680	680	680	mW
temperature (see Note 5)	L Package	625	625	625	
Operating free-air temperature range		−55 to 125	−25 to 85	0 to 70	°C
Storage temperature range		−65 to 150	−65 to 150	−65 to 150	°C
Lead temperature 1/16 inch from case for 60 seconds	J, JG, or L Package	300	300	300	°C
Lead temperature 1/16 inch from case for 10 seconds	N or P Package		260	260	°C

NOTES:
1. All voltage values, except differential voltages, are with respect to the zero reference level (ground) of the supply voltages where the zero reference level is the midpoint between V_{CC+} and V_{CC-}.
2. Differential voltages are at the noninverting input terminal with respect to the inverting input terminal.
3. The magnitude of the input voltage must never exceed the magnitude of the supply voltage or 15 volts, whichever is less.
4. The output may be shorted to ground or to either supply. Temperature and/or supply voltages must be limited to ensure that the dissipation rating is not exceeded.
5. For operation above 25°C free-air temperature, refer to Dissipation Derating Table.

DISSIPATION DERATING TABLE

PACKAGE	POWER RATING	DERATING FACTOR	ABOVE T_A
J	680 mW	8.2 mW/°C	67°C
JG	680 mW	6.6 mW/°C	47°C
L	625 mW	5.0 mW/°C	25°C
N	680 mW	9.2 mW/°C	76°C
P	680 mW	8.0 mW/°C	65°C

DEVICE TYPES, SUFFIX VERSIONS, AND PACKAGES

	TL070	TL071	TL072	TL074	TL075
TL07_M	JG,L	JG,L	JG,L	J	*
TL07_I	JG,L,P	JG,L,P	JG,L,P	J,N	*
TL07_C	JG,L,P	JG,L,P	JG,L,P	J,N	N
TL07_AC	JG,L,P	JG,L,P	JG,L,P	J,N	*
TL07_BC	*	JG,L,P	JG,L,P	J,N	*

*These combinations are not defined by this data sheet.

electrical characteristics, $V_{CC\pm} = \pm 15$ V

PARAMETER		TEST CONDITIONS†		TL07_M MIN	TYP	MAX	TL07_I MIN	TYP	MAX	TL07_C TL07_AC TL07_BC MIN	TYP	MAX	UNIT
V_{IO} Input offset voltage	$R_S = 50\ \Omega$, $T_A = 25^\circ C$		'70, '71, '72, '75‡		3	6		3	6		3	10	mV
			'74		3	9		3	6		3	10	
			'70A, '71A, '72A, '74A								3	6	
			'71B, '72B, '74B								2	3	
	$R_S = 50\ \Omega$, $T_A = $ full range		'70, '71, '72, '75‡			9			9			13	
			'74			15			9			13	
			'70A, '71A, '72A, '74A									7.5	
			'71B, '72B, '74B									5	
α_{VIO} Temperature coefficient of input offset voltage	$R_S = 50\ \Omega$,	$T_A = $ full range			10			10			10		$\mu V/^\circ C$
I_{IO} Input offset current§	$T_A = 25^\circ C$		'70, '71, '72, '74, '75‡		5	50		5	50		5	50	pA
			'70A, '71A, '72A, '74A								5	50	
			'71B, '72B, '74B								5	50	
	$T_A = $ full range		'70, '71, '72, '74, '75‡			20			10			2	nA
			'70A, '71A, '72A, '74A									2	
			'71B, '72B, '74B									2	
I_{IB} Input bias current§	$T_A = 25^\circ C$		'70, '71, '72, '74, '75‡		30	200		30	200		30	200	pA
			'70A, '71A, '72A, '74A								30	200	
			'71B, '72B, '74B								30	200	
	$T_A = $ full range		'70, '71, '72, '74, '75‡			50			20			7	nA
			'70A, '71A, '72A, '74A									7	
			'71B, '72B, '74B									7	
V_{ICR} Common-mode input voltage range	$T_A = 25^\circ C$		'70, '71, '72, '74, '75‡	±12			±12			±10			V
			'70A, '71A, '72A, '74A							±12			
			'71B, '72B, '74B							±12			
V_{OPP} Maximum peak-to-peak output voltage swing	$T_A = 25^\circ C$,	$R_L = 10\ k\Omega$		24	27		24	27		24	27		V
	$T_A = $ full range	$R_L \geqslant 10\ k\Omega$		24			24			24			
		$R_L \geqslant 2\ k\Omega$		20	24		20	24		20	24		
A_{VD} Large-signal differential voltage amplification	$R_L \geqslant 2\ k\Omega$, $V_O = \pm 10$ V, $T_A = 25^\circ C$		'70, '71, '72, '74, '75‡	50	200		50	200		25	200		V/mV
			'70A, '71A, '72A, '74A							50	200		
			'71B, '72B, '74B							50	200		
	$R_L \geqslant 2\ k\Omega$, $V_O = \pm 10$ V, $T_A = $ full range		'70, '71, '72, '74, '75‡	25			25			15			
			'70A, '71A, '72A, '74A							25			
			'71B, '72B, '74B							25			
B_1 Unity-gain bandwidth	$T_A = 25^\circ C$,	$R_L = 10\ k\Omega$			3			3			3		MHz
r_i Input resistance	$T_A = 25^\circ C$				10^{12}			10^{12}			10^{12}		Ω
CMRR Common-mode rejection ratio	$R_S \leqslant 10\ k\Omega$, $T_A = 25^\circ C$		'70, '71, '72, '74, '75‡	80	86		80	86		70	76		dB
			'70A, '71A, '72A, '74A							80	86		
			'71B, '72B, '74B							80	86		
k_{SVR} Supply voltage rejection ratio ($\Delta V_{CC\pm}/\Delta V_{IO}$)	$R_S \leqslant 10\ k\Omega$, $T_A = 25^\circ C$		'70, '71, '72, '74, '75‡	80	86		80	86		70	76		dB
			'70A, '71A, '72A, '74A							80	86		
			'71B, '72B, '74B							80	86		
I_{CC} Supply current (per amplifier)	No load, $T_A = 25^\circ C$	No signal,			1.4	2.5		1.4	2.5		1.4	2.5	mA
V_{o1}/V_{o2} Channel separation	$A_{VD} = 100$,	$T_A = 25^\circ C$			120			120			120		dB

†All characteristics are specified under open-loop conditions unless otherwise noted. Full range for T_A is $-55^\circ C$ to $125^\circ C$ for TL07_M; $-25^\circ C$ to $85^\circ C$ for TL07_I; and $0^\circ C$ to $70^\circ C$ for TL07_C, TL07_AC, and TL07_BC.

‡Types TL075I and TL075M are not defined by this data sheet.

§Input bias currents of a FET-input operational amplifier are normal junction reverse currents, which are temperature sensitive as shown in Figure 18. Pulse techniques must be used that will maintain the junction temperatures as close to the ambient temperature as is possible.

TYPES TL070, TL070A, TL071, TL071A, TL071B, TL072, TL072A, TL072B, TL074, TL074A, TL074B, TL075
LOW-NOISE JFET-INPUT OPERATIONAL AMPLIFIERS

operating characteristics, $V_{CC\pm} = \pm 15$ V, $T_A = 25°C$

	PARAMETER	TEST CONDITIONS		MIN	TYP	MAX	UNIT
SR	Slew rate at unity gain	$V_I = 10$ V, $C_L = 100$ pF,	$R_L = 2$ kΩ, See Figure 1		13		V/μs
t_r	Rise time	$V_I = 20$ mV, $C_L = 100$ pF,	$R_L = 2$ kΩ, See Figure 1		0.1		μs
	Overshoot factor				10%		
V_n	Equivalent input noise voltage	$R_S = 100$ Ω	f = 1 kHz		18		nV/$\sqrt{Hz}$
			f = 10 Hz to 10 kHz		4		μV
I_n	Equivalent input noise current	$R_S = 100$ Ω,	f = 1 kHz		0.01		pA/$\sqrt{Hz}$
THD	Total harmonic distortion	$V_{O(rms)} = 10$ V, $R_L \geqslant 2$ kΩ,	$R_S \leqslant 1$ kΩ, f = 1 kHz		0.01%		

PARAMETER MEASUREMENT INFORMATION

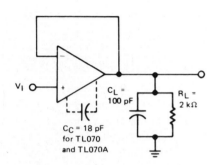

FIGURE 1—UNITY-GAIN AMPLIFIER

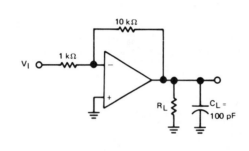

FIGURE 2—GAIN-OF-10 INVERTING AMPLIFIER

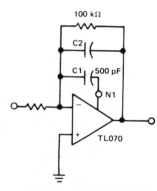

FIGURE 3—FEED-FORWARD COMPENSATION

INPUT OFFSET VOLTAGE NULL CIRCUITS

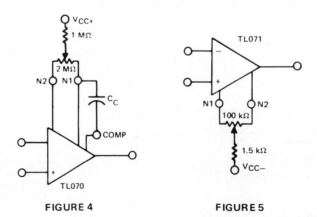

FIGURE 4

FIGURE 5

TYPICAL CHARACTERISTICS†

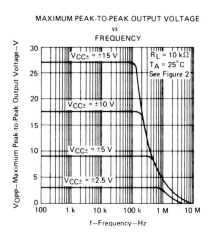

MAXIMUM PEAK-TO-PEAK OUTPUT VOLTAGE
vs
FREQUENCY

FIGURE 6

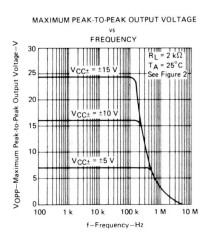

MAXIMUM PEAK-TO-PEAK OUTPUT VOLTAGE
vs
FREQUENCY

FIGURE 7

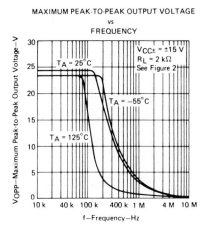

MAXIMUM PEAK-TO-PEAK OUTPUT VOLTAGE
vs
FREQUENCY

FIGURE 8

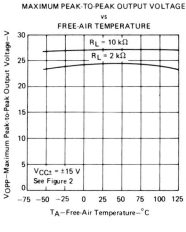

MAXIMUM PEAK-TO-PEAK OUTPUT VOLTAGE
vs
FREE-AIR TEMPERATURE

FIGURE 9

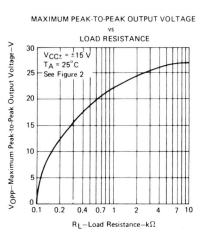

MAXIMUM PEAK-TO-PEAK OUTPUT VOLTAGE
vs
LOAD RESISTANCE

FIGURE 10

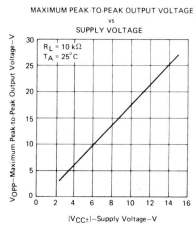

MAXIMUM PEAK-TO-PEAK OUTPUT VOLTAGE
vs
SUPPLY VOLTAGE

FIGURE 11

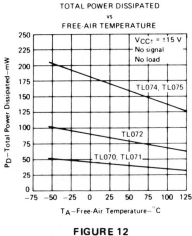

TOTAL POWER DISSIPATED
vs
FREE-AIR TEMPERATURE

FIGURE 12

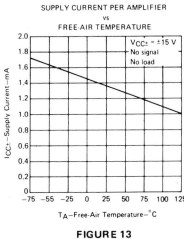

SUPPLY CURRENT PER AMPLIFIER
vs
FREE-AIR TEMPERATURE

FIGURE 13

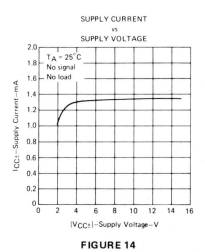

SUPPLY CURRENT
vs
SUPPLY VOLTAGE

FIGURE 14

†Data at high and low temperatures are applicable only within the rated operating free-air temperature ranges of the various devices. A 18-pF compensation capacitor is used with TL070 and TL070A.

TYPICAL CHARACTERISTICS†

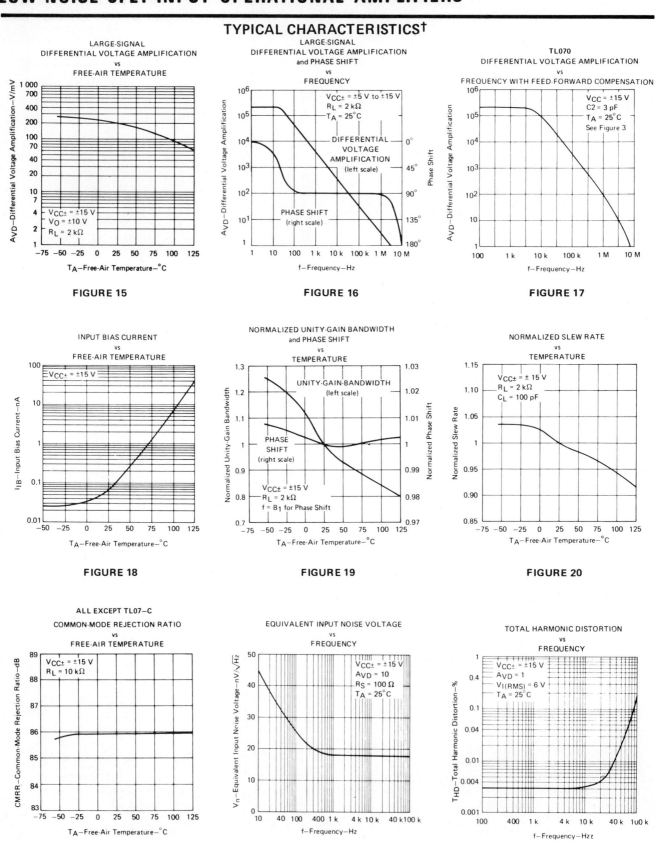

FIGURE 15

FIGURE 16

FIGURE 17

FIGURE 18

FIGURE 19

FIGURE 20

FIGURE 21

FIGURE 22

FIGURE 23

†Data at high and low temperatures are applicable only within the rated operating free-air temperature ranges of the various devices. A 18-pF compensation capacitor is used with TL070 and TL070A.

TYPICAL CHARACTERISTICS†

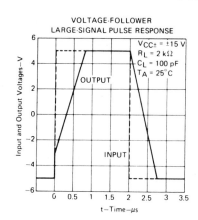

VOLTAGE-FOLLOWER
LARGE-SIGNAL PULSE RESPONSE

$V_{CC\pm} = \pm15$ V
$R_L = 2$ kΩ
$C_L = 100$ pF
$T_A = 25°C$

FIGURE 24

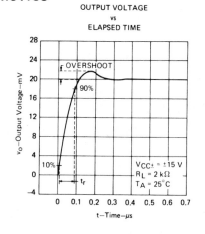

OUTPUT VOLTAGE
vs
ELAPSED TIME

$V_{CC\pm} = \pm15$ V
$R_L = 2$ kΩ
$T_A = 25°C$

FIGURE 25

†Data at high and low temperatures are applicable only within the rated operating free-air temperature ranges of the various devices. A 18-pF compensation capacitor is used with TL070 and TL070A.

TYPICAL APPLICATION DATA

0.5-Hz SQUARE-WAVE OSCILLATOR

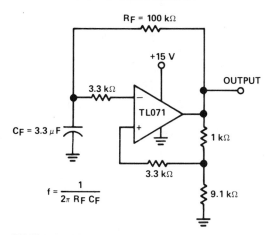

$R_F = 100$ kΩ

$C_F = 3.3 \mu F$

$f = \dfrac{1}{2\pi R_F C_F}$

FIGURE 26—0.5-Hz SQUARE-WAVE OSCILLATOR

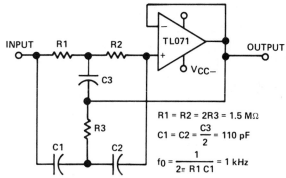

$R1 = R2 = 2R3 = 1.5$ MΩ

$C1 = C2 = \dfrac{C3}{2} = 110$ pF

$f_0 = \dfrac{1}{2\pi R1\, C1} = 1$ kHz

FIGURE 27—HIGH-Q NOTCH FILTER

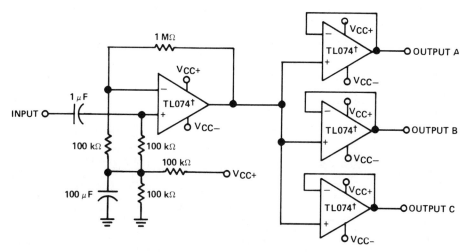

† or TL075

FIGURE 28—AUDIO DISTRIBUTION AMPLIFIER

TYPICAL APPLICATION DATA

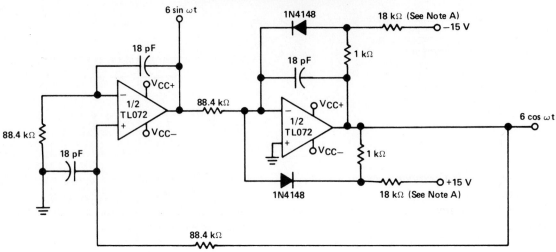

Note A: These resistor values may be adjusted for a symmetrical output.

FIGURE 29—100-KHz QUADRATURE OSCILLATOR

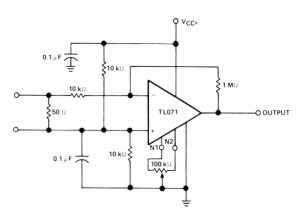

FIGURE 30—AC AMPLIFIER

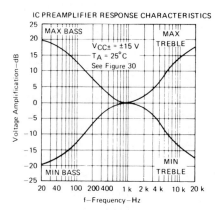

IC PREAMPLIFIER RESPONSE CHARACTERISTICS

$V_{CC\pm} = \pm15$ V
$T_A = 25°C$
See Figure 30

FIGURE 31

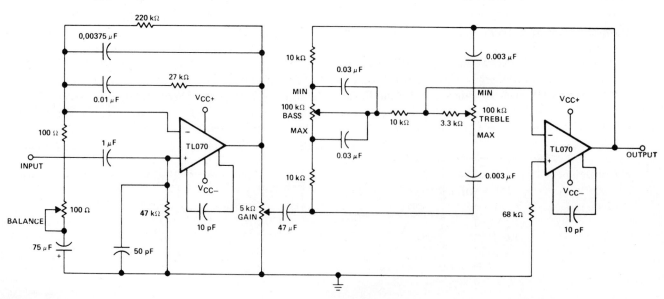

FIGURE 32--IC PREAMPLIFIER

Bibliography

Applications Manual for Operational Amplifiers, Philbrick/Nexur, Dedham, Mass.

Biomedical Instrumentation, Marvin D. Weiss, Chilton, Philadelphia.

A Case Book of Basic Circuits for Electronics Instrumentation, George C. Stanley, Jr., 1971. Rinehart, San Francisco, Calif.

Data Book for Electronic Technicians and Engineers, John D. Lenk, Prentice-Hall, Englewood Cliffs, N.J.

Designing Circuits with I.C. Operational Amplifiers, Robert G. Seippel, American Technical Society, Chicago, Ill.

Digital Electronics for Scientists, Malmstadt, Enke, W.A. Benjamin, Inc. N.Y.

Electronic Troubleshooting, Clyde N. Herrick, Reston Publishing, Reston, Vir.

General Instrument Corp., Microelectronics Division, Hicksville N.Y.

Handbook of Electronic Charts, Graphs and Tables, John D. Lenk, Prentice-Hall, Englewood Cliffs, NJ.

Handbook of I.C. Circuit Projects, Jim Ashe, Tab Books, Blue Ridge Summit, Penn.

Handbook of Oscilloscopes, John D. Lenk, Prentice-Hall, Englewood Cliffs, N.J.

Handbook of Telemetry, Elliot L. Greenberg, McGraw-Hill, N.Y.

How to Build and Use Electronic Devices Without Frustration, Panic, Mountains of Money, or an Engineering Degree—Stuart A. Hoenig and F. Leland Payne, Little, Brown, Boston.

I. C. Op-Amp Cookbook, Walter Jung, Bobbs—Merrill, Indianapolis.

Integrated Circuits Catalog for Design Engineers, Texas Instruments, Inc., Dallas, TX.

Integrated Electronics, Millman and Halkias, McGraw-Hill, N.Y.

Introduction to Medical Electronics, Burton R. Klein, Tab Books, Blue Ridge Summit, Penn.

Linear Applications, vols. 1 and 2, National Semiconductor Corp., Santa Clara, Calif.

Linear Data Book, June 1976, National Semiconductor Corp., Santa Clara, Calif.

Linear Integrated Circuits, J. Eimbinder, Wiley, N.Y.

Linear Integrated Circuits, vol. 6, ser. A, 1975, Motorola Semiconductor Products, Phoenix, Ariz.

Linear Integrated Circuits Data Catalog, Fairchild Instrument Corp. Mountain View, Calif.

Linear Integrated Circuits, I.C.-42 RCA, Somerville, N.J.

Measurement Systems, Application and Design, E.O. Doeblin, McGraw-Hill, N.Y.

Modern Applications of Linear IC's, Tab Books, Blue Ridge Summit, Penn.

Nonlinear Circuits Handbook, Engineering Staff of Analog Devices, Inc., Norwood, Mass. 1974

111 Digital and Linear I.C. Projects, Don Tuite, Tab Books, Blue Ridge Summit, Penn.

OP AMP Circuit Design & Applications, Joseph Carr, Tab Books, Blue Ridge Summit, Penn.

Operational Amplifiers, Tobey, Graeme, Huelsman, McGraw-Hill, N.Y. 1971

Phaselocked Loop Design Fundamentals, AN-535, Motorola Semiconductor Products, Box 20912, Phoenix, Ariz.

Phaselock Techniques, Floyd M. Gardner, Wiley, N.Y.

Principles of Coherent Communication, Andrew Viterb, McGraw-Hill, N.Y.

Signetics, Digital, Linear, MOS Applications, Signetics Corp., Sunnyvale, Calif.

Signetics, Digital, Linear, MOS Data Book, Signetics Corp., Sunnyvale, Calif.

Solid State Devices 5C-16, RCA, Somerville, N.J.